Ma del Socorro Martinez Becerra
Juan Armando Flores D.
Alejandra Jimenez Diaz

Main routine clinical tests in a Clinical Laboratory

Ma del Socorro Martinez Becerra
Juan Armando Flores D.
Alejandra Jimenez Diaz

Main routine clinical tests in a Clinical Laboratory

Clinical Laboratory tools for disease diagnosis

ScienciaScripts

Imprint

Any brand names and product names mentioned in this book are subject to trademark, brand or patent protection and are trademarks or registered trademarks of their respective holders. The use of brand names, product names, common names, trade names, product descriptions etc. even without a particular marking in this work is in no way to be construed to mean that such names may be regarded as unrestricted in respect of trademark and brand protection legislation and could thus be used by anyone.

Cover image: www.ingimage.com

This book is a translation from the original published under ISBN 978-613-9-41022-4.

Publisher:
Sciencia Scripts
is a trademark of
Dodo Books Indian Ocean Ltd. and OmniScriptum S.R.L publishing group

120 High Road, East Finchley, London, N2 9ED, United Kingdom
Str. Armeneasca 28/1, office 1, Chisinau MD-2012, Republic of Moldova, Europe
Printed at: see last page
ISBN: 978-620-6-52180-8

Table of Contents

To my parents who have followed my every step, because I recognize the great effort and sacrifice they have made for me and my siblings.

1. Objectives

1.1 Overall objective

Describe in detail the procedures of the tests that are performed in a clinical laboratory, in order to generate results that are completely reliable.

Always guaranteeing quality results, accurate and reliable analytical data in a timely manner and at acceptable costs for the patients who come to the clinical analysis laboratory.

1.2 Specific objectives

- Describe the areas that make up the laboratory.

- Describe each of the procedures carried out in the laboratory from the moment the patient arrives until the results are delivered.

- To make known the analyses performed and their clinical usefulness.

2. Mission, Vision and Values

2.1 Mission

To provide a service of clinical analysis, reliable and timely, auxiliary in the diagnosis of clinical pathologies, on a basis of professional ethics and high commitment to improving the quality of life of the population. Always with the highest technological professional development and improvement in the warmth of its service.

2.2 Vision

To provide information on a wide variety of specialized and high quality studies to physicians and patients, making us the leader in medicine with our primary objective of making the clinical laboratory the preferred laboratory for excellence in quality and service.

2.3 Values that a clinical laboratory should have

- Ethics
- Honesty
- Quality
- Responsibility
- Honesty
- Kindness
- Discretion

3. Introduction

The pharmaceutical chemist-biologist in the laboratory performs clinical analysis or tests that consist of the study of the components of biological samples taken from the patient such as blood, urine, feces, tissue. Where their results are of valuable utility to confirm or rule out a medical diagnosis, as well as to monitor the effect of a given treatment.

The usefulness of clinical analysis is not restricted only to sick people who must be diagnosed, since a periodic check-up in healthy people from 6 to 12 months is very important in the form of prevention, for the detection of various ailments, especially those of chronic type, which at first do not generate symptoms, such as diabetes, hypertension and cancer among others, and early, allowing to prevent their evolution and maintaining a good state of health.

We can consider that the laboratory is the place where clinical analyses are performed that contribute to the study, prevention, diagnosis and treatment of patients' health problems.

Clinical analyses are indispensable for the physician, since they provide him with the necessary information for the resolution of a diagnostic problem, as well as the elements of judgment to consider the importance of the phenomena, and above all, to objectively support the prognosis of a disease; they also give him a safe orientation about the therapy and follow-up of the same that allow him to have the necessary elements in the evaluation of the state of health in the population.

The pharmaceutical chemist-biologist must know the methods and techniques for the processing of biological material, how to obtain samples, as well as constantly updating his scientific and clinical knowledge necessary to be an active part of the ambulatory and hospital care teams.

It also assists in the diagnosis through the interpretation of both normal and pathological results. Always taking care of the guidelines according to the sensitivity, specificity, precision, and the current regulations of the laboratory.

A clinical laboratory can provide services to the community and can be integrated by the following areas:

- Reception and waiting room

- Administrative area

- Sampling

- Hematology and coagulation

- Blood chemistry

- Serology

- General urine test

4. Location

The location of a laboratory is of utmost importance as this is one of the key pieces to be able to be the first options to what corresponds to the comfort that is provided to the patient or the doctor in your case.

5. Organization chart

By means of the following organization chart we can observe the hierarchies of each of the members that make up a clinical laboratory.

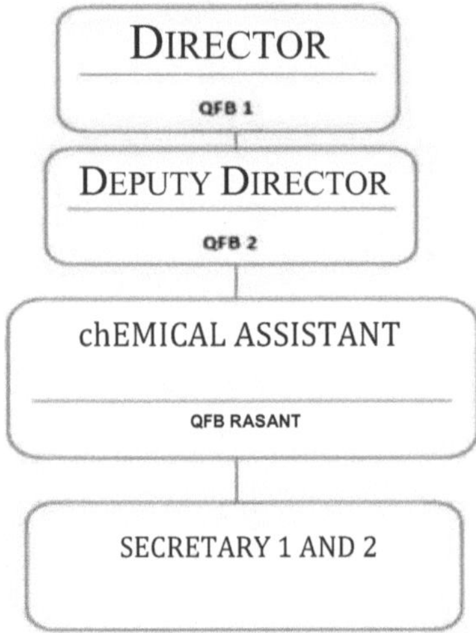

Figure 1. Hierarchical organization chart of the personnel working in the Laboratory

The personnel working in the laboratory perform the following functions:

5.1 Director

- Laboratory responsibility

- Technical and administrative authority of financial resources (purchase of reagents, materials and supplies for the laboratory).

- Supervising (sample taking, analytical methods, human relations)

- Evaluate the technical capacity of personnel

- Monitor the correct operation and maintenance of the equipment.

- Coordinate staff substitutions

5.2 Deputy Director

- Communicating serious misconduct to management

- Work scheduling

- Reagent orders from different areas

- Calibration and reagent preparation

- Equipment handling

- Examinations

- Interpretation of results

5.3 Chemistry Assistant

- Execute orders from management and management.

- Inform the patient about the conditions according to the requested study.

- Sampling

- Sample preparation

- Support in handling equipment

5.4 Secretaries who may vary their jobs depending on the laboratory

- Equipment start-up and material preparation

- Patient care by taking personal data and receiving medical requests.

- Cash receipts

- Recording and filling of the computation system

- Worksheets elaboration

- Tagged

- Pouring and delivery of results report

- Distribution of materials and reagents

- Laboratory cleaning

- Material washing

- Preparation of inventory of inputs

6. Laboratory layout

The laboratory can be distributed in three different spaces, below is a scheme that allows us to understand how they are located. The mentioned areas will be described chronologically.

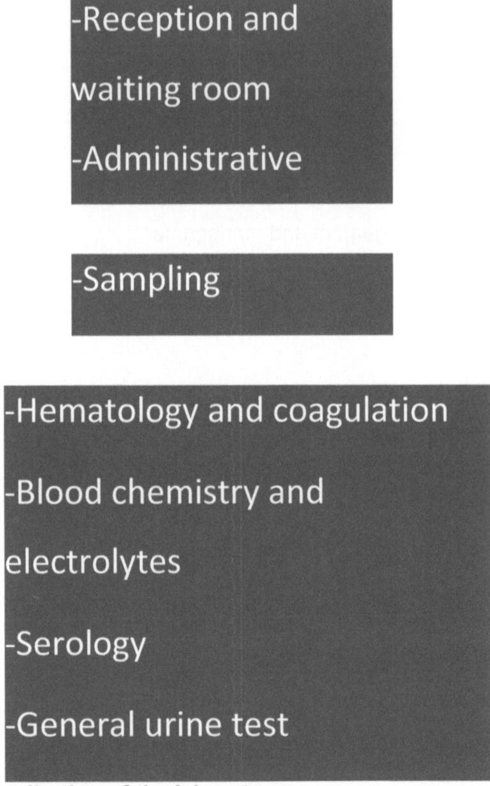

Figure 2. Spatial distribution of the laboratory.

7. Reception and waiting room

7.1 Reception

The reception area is located at the entrance of the laboratory, where the staff initially receives patients and provides them with the necessary information. In this area different functions are performed, such as:

7.1.1 Patient reception

•   Reception of outpatients with orders for analysis.

Immediately the medical orders are entered into the laboratory's computer system and then taken to the sample reception area, where they are filled out manually and marked for labeling, and the samples are placed in the corresponding racks.

•   Patients are received according to their appointments.

•   Information is provided on the cost of the tests to be performed.

•   Receive samples that were taken in advance at the health care facility, their homes or at the community hospital.

•   Collect your personal data to enter them into the system.

•   Give precise instructions on the conditions under which the patient must present himself/herself to obtain the sample.

7.1.2 General indications for blood sampling

1.   The ideal fasting period is 8 hours, only for some tests.

2.   For lipid profile a fasting period of 10 to 12 hours is requested. Avoiding the consumption of meals with high fat content 24 hours before.

3.   For coagulation tests, do not take the anticoagulant in the morning until after the sample has been taken.

4.   Do not drink alcoholic beverages 24 hours before.

5.   Do not smoke before performing the examinations.

6.   Avoid exercising the day before the exams.

7.   You must inform if you are a diabetic patient.

8.   Inform if you are taking any type of medication, as well as the possible diagnosis suggested by the physician.

7.1.3 Indications for General Urine Test

1.   The first urine of the morning is requested in a bottle provided by the laboratory.

2.   When the patient does not carry urine, he/she is asked to collect the specimen in a laboratory container when the urine has been in his/her bladder for 2 to 3 hours.

3.   Discard the initial stream of urine and collect only the intermediate stream in the bottle. It should be filled approximately halfway and never to the top.

4.   Female patients should use very clean fingers to open the genital lips and hold them apart when collecting the sample into the bottle. If you are on your menstrual period, please notify us. Male patients, if uncircumcised, will need to retract the foreskin first.

7.1.4 Indications for 24-hour urine collection

1.   A 5 liter container is provided for sample collection.

2.   The collection begins by urinating, emptying the bladder, and that urine is flushed down the toilet.

3.   From this moment on, all 24-hour urine should be collected (keep refrigerated) and the time of the first collection should be noted.

4.   At the completion of exactly 24 hours, this urine will be added to the previously collected urine and the entire volume will be delivered to the laboratory in less than two hours.

5.   If urine is lost during collection, throw the urine away and start again from the beginning.

6.   The weight and height of the patient should be reported to the laboratory.

7.1.5 Preliminary indications for microbiological sampling for Upper Respiratory Infection

1.   Come to the laboratory fasting without oral hygiene.

2.   Do not use mouthwash on the day of sampling.

3.   Do not smoke before or during sampling.

4.   Do not drink alcoholic beverages three days before the test.

5.   If you are taking any medication, you must notify us.

It is a very frequent specimen taken to the laboratory. Collection of urine for urine culture can be done in the laboratory or at home (it should be taken within 1-2 hours of collection).

The technique used is spontaneous urination, the sample is collected after cleaning the genitals properly with benzal, for the collection must use sterile container, cover without touching the edges of it, discard the first portion of urine and collect 5-15mL of the remaining volume, discarding the final stream.

The procedure for women consists of separating the labia by wiping the area with benzal and placing the middle stream of urine in the bottle.

For men, it consists of disinfecting with benzal, starting with the urethral area, making outward movements of the head of the penis with the previous retention of the foreskin, in the same way to collect the middle stream of urine.

If the patient is taking antibiotics, he/she should wait five days after finishing the treatment to undergo the test.

7.2 Waiting room

The waiting room is a large space with adequate lighting and ventilation, which is located at the entrance of the laboratory. Where the patient waits for his or her turn to enter the sample taking area and for the delivery of results.

8. Administrative area

It is a very important physical area of the laboratory and should be located at the entrance of the laboratory to facilitate communication with outsiders who consult with him. It has an adequate dimension to serve the public, it is the place for desk work, it has a file cabinet, telephone line and extension to answer calls in any area of the laboratory (1).

The administrative area is used to carry out the following:

1.   The filling out of personal data of each patient such as age, sex, date of birth, studies to be performed, to whom they are addressed, telephone number, address, etc.

2.   Receipt of requests for laboratory tests.

3.   Elaboration of worksheets. These worksheets are prepared for distribution to the different areas or sections. They indicate the identification of the sample, its order of priority, and the requested determinations. They are given to the chemists and laboratory assistants so that they can perform the analytical determinations requested for each patient. All in order to work in the most clear and precise way.

4.   Elaboration of the results reports. It consists of filling in the results obtained from each patient after analytical processing.

After the chemists perform the analytical determinations, the results obtained are entered into the computer system for each patient. They consist of numerical values and signs to show the pathological values, as well as reference values for each analyte.

Reports are usually sent electronically via the Internet to both physicians and patients, who can access the laboratory's historical archive for consultation when necessary. For this purpose, passwords are assigned to them, so that only authorized personnel can access the results.

5.   Printing of the results to be delivered.

6.   Advance payments made prior to delivery.

9. Sampling area

Samples are taken here and then distributed to the various sections of the laboratory.

9.1 Venous blood collection

To obtain the patient's blood in the laboratory, samples are taken from the forearm, by means of a venous puncture.

Venous puncture allows a greater amount of blood to be drawn for the necessary tests required by the laboratory. The veins of choice are those on the anterior aspect of the forearm (cubital vein, cephalic vein and basilic vein) because they are much easier to access.

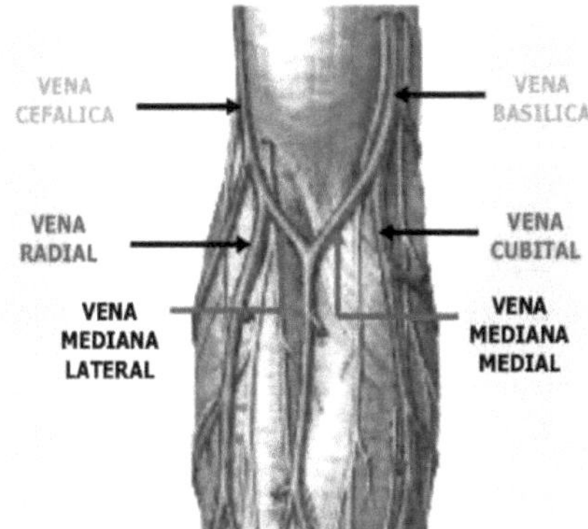

Figure 3. Forearm veins used for phlebotomy.

9.1.1 Pre-puncture considerations

- Avoid puncturing in an area where there is skin damage.

- If there are difficulties to extract the sample, the extremity is warmed with massages. The extremity should be allowed to remain tilted for several minutes before the puncture is performed.

9.1.2 Patient preparation and extraction methodology

- Ask the patient to take a seat by instructing him/her to place his/her arm on the table.

- Instruct the patient on the technique for taking the sample.

- Mention that the needle insertion will be painful.

- Prepare the material to be used, Vacutainer tubes, swabs, tourniquet, syringes, slides to perform the smear.

- The patient is asked to uncover both arms.

- Fully extend the arm with the palmar surface upward. With the patient's help.

- Place the tourniquet on the upper arm (approximately 5 cm above the crease) to produce venous congestion. Prolonged tourniquet causes stasis and hemo-concentration. The loop should be placed so as to produce a compression of the muscle no greater than 1 mm.

- Select the puncture site: Ask the patient to open and close the puncture several times; choose an accessible vein.

- Disinfect the area with an alcohol swab and wait for it to dry.

- To perform the puncture the patient must have the puncture closed.

- Place the tip of the needle at an angle of 15-30° over the surface of the chosen vein and pass through the skin with a firm and steady movement, all the way to the lumen of the vein.

- Once the vein is penetrated, the syringe is filled by pulling the plunger in a continuous motion to draw blood up to the required volume.

- Ask the patient to open the puncture and loosen the tourniquet so that the blood flows better, then remove the needle from the arm with a gentle movement. At the end of the collection, place a cotton swab on the puncture area.

- Press the cotton to avoid hematoma formation, waiting for it to coagulate.

- Discard needles and/or syringes in an appropriate container.

- The Vacutainer tubes are filled up to the mark indicated.

- A blood smear is performed.

- Once the bleeding stops, the patient is asked to return for the results in a couple of hours.

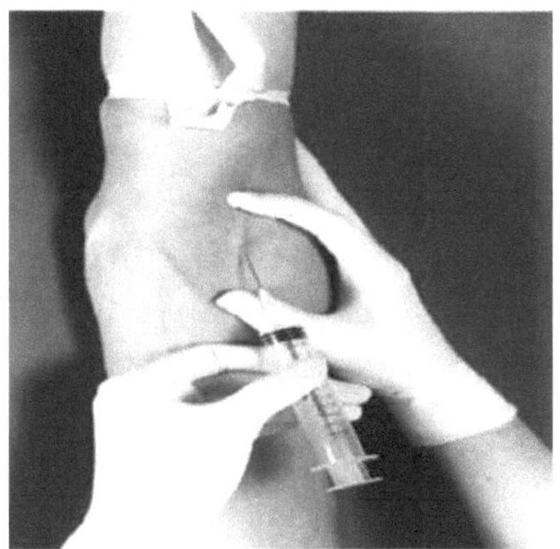

Figure 4. Obtaining venous blood from the forearm, the most common technique used in the laboratory.

9.1.3 General precautions

The strictest standards of hygiene must be observed during sampling. Practicing the minimum universal precautions with every patient to be treated. All samples should be considered potentially infectious and precautions should be taken to ensure the safety of the chemist and patients. At all times hair should be kept up, in addition to wearing a lab coat, taking care to use disposable gloves during the extraction, which will be kept on during the entire procedure, if they become filled with any fluid change them immediately and clean the area with 10% sodium hypochlorite.

9.2 Microbiological sampling

Obtaining these samples is a specialized procedure that consists of obtaining biological specimens in order to isolate, incubate and determine which agents are responsible for an infection.

9.2.1 Upper Respiratory Infection Sample Collection

Throat swab: Lower the tongue and rub the tonsils, anterior pillars and posterior pharyngeal wall with the sterile swab. Place in the transport medium and send immediately to the laboratory, if not possible the sample is kept temporarily at room temperature.

The correct method of obtaining a pharyngeal swab sample is shown in Figure 6. A bright light should be shone into the oral cavity, over the shoulder of the person taking the sample, so as to bring the swab to the posterior pharynx. The patient is instructed to tilt his or her head back and take a deep breath. The tongue is gently pressed with a tongue bat to visualize the tonsillar fossae and posterior pharynx. The swab is extended between the tonsillar pillars behind the uvula. Care should be taken not to touch the lateral walls of the oral cavity or the tongue to minimize contamination with commensal bacteria. When the patient pronounces a long "ah", it facilitates the allocution of the umbilicus and helps to avoid gagging. The tonsillar areas and the back of the pharynx should be firmly swabbed with the swab. Any purulent exudate should be sampled (2).

After collection, the swab should be placed immediately into a sterile tube or other suitable container for transport to the laboratory.

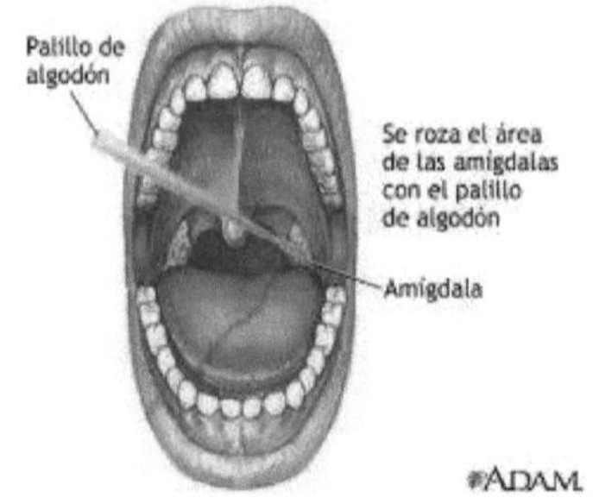

Figure 5. Pharyngeal culture technique.

9.3 Identification, distribution, processing and storage

9.3.1 Identification

At all times it is important to identify the samples, as the reliability of the personnel who obtain or collect them depends on this. In the containers where the samples are placed there is a previous labeling and marking, where in a white label the full name, age, sex, and the request number that is assigned to identify the patient are written.

9.3.2 Distribution

The sample distribution process must be very well organized, otherwise it can be the source of numerous errors. An important aspect of the samples is their handling, which includes the separation of the caps from the tubes and the aliquoting to the different sections of the laboratory. All this processing is done with latex gloves. When preparing the aliquots and distributing the samples, it is essential to do it carefully, to avoid errors and to avoid interchanging specimens and/or mixing them. It is very important to identify well the secondary containers and to use disposable pipettes, one for each patient or sample.

9.3.3 processing

Once the blood sample is obtained, the blood is placed in the different tubes, depending on the study that is intended to be performed is the processing that will be given to the sample.

The Vacutainer tubes used in the laboratory are classified in different cap colors, depending on the color indicates the additive or absence of the same contained in the tube. Something very important to mention is that the tubes contain added substances to preserve the blood, to avoid alteration of the hemolytes, not to produce hemolysis, to avoid platelet aggregation and not to alter the morphology of the leukocytes.

The additive and use contained in each of the tubes is as follows:

Serum. Serum plastic tubes have coagulation activator, and are used for serum determinations in clinical chemistry and serology.

Serum with separating gel. They contain coagulation activator and a serum separating polymer gel. They are used for serum and clinical chemistry determinations.

Citrate. With citrate for regular testing of clotting times. The clinical advantages they have are the sodium citrate concentrations that can have significant effects on TTP and PT tests.

EDTA. EDTA tubes are used for hematological determinations with whole blood (3).

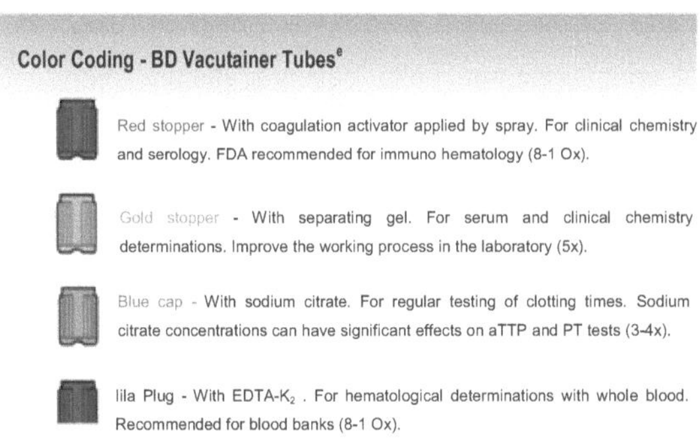

The proper order for filling the tubes is as follows:

1.   The first tube to be filled is the blood culture tube (if that test is ordered).

2.   Tubes without additive, as is the case of the red cap for chemistry and serology.

3.   The tubes with gold or yellow separating gel used in the determination of blood chemistry.

4.   The light blue coagulation test tubes should never be the first ones, being quickly mixed after being taken.

5.   The following tubes are those used to avoid coagulation, which would be lilac or purple in color. They should still be quickly mixed immediately after being taken.

The tubes with anticoagulant should be gently inverted 8 times to homogenize properly, always taking care of the correct mixture of the additives of the tube with the blood sample, it is important to fill it up to the indicated mark to avoid that the concentration of the anticoagulant is too high. The tubes that do not contain anticoagulant should not be moved to avoid hemolysis, and they should be centrifuged 30 minutes after the extraction of the sample (4).

Immediately after filling all the tubes and before discarding the syringe, the blood smear is performed on the slide, a method of utmost importance for the microscopic description of blood biometry. This process will be described in depth in the area of hematology and coagulation.

The next step is to gather a considerable amount of samples, the tubes that are subjected to centrifugation are those containing red, yellow and light blue cap; Since from here a quota will be taken to be analyzed, In the laboratory a speed of 4000 revolutions per minute is used in a period of time of 5 minutes separating the plasma from the globular package. The samples should not be centrifuged again after obtaining the plasma.

The tubes are distributed to the corresponding areas of the laboratory for specific analysis, if any:

<u>Lilac or purple colored cap tube</u>. Area of hematology and coagulation, where before being processed by means of the clitometer it is homogenized in the hematological mixer of tubes for biometry.

<u>Light blue colored cap tube</u>. Coagulation area, where part of the plasma is taken for its previous analysis.

<u>Yellow or gold colored cap tube</u>. Area of blood chemistry and serology.

<u>Red colored cap tube.</u> These samples are sent to reference laboratories for more expensive and specific tests.

The laboratory should have extensive studies, if it does not have the infrastructure should be sought to be channeled to specialized laboratories, for this aliquots of blood plasma are taken in marked eppendorf tubes, urine cultures are marked and refrigerated upon delivery, along with the throat swab sample are transported in refrigerator to the aforementioned destination.

The vast majority of the samples analyzed in the laboratory is blood, where it is defined as a red colored fluid with a viscous appearance, composed of plasma and different formed elements, where 45-50% is made up of cells (erythrocytes, leukocytes and platelets) and 50-55% is plasma, where 90% is water and only the remaining 10% are the different dissolved substances such as proteins, enzymes, electrolytes or waste substances.

These cells originate from a single cell called stem cell which is found in the hematopoietic organs and can mature into any of these three cell types. Once their maturation is completed, the cells pass into the general circulation, where after a certain time, they are eliminated, thus maintaining the constant renewal of the elements that constitute the blood (5).

In the case of other biological liquids such as urine, doctors consider the general urine test a very basic study and of utmost importance for a given diagnosis, the samples are found in smaller quantities in the laboratory, where the processing for the realization consists of homogenizing the sample, using a centrifuge speed of 4000 rpm for a period of 4 minutes.

9.3.4 Storage

The laboratory has a refrigerator, the remnants of serum and blood plasma are refrigerated once all processing is completed, only in case patients are subsequently requested for further analytical determinations. Storage is for approximately eight days at a temperature between 2-8°C.

10.Hematology and coagulation

The area of hematology and coagulation is so fundamental that it is considered probably the most frequently requested laboratory study, along with general urinalysis and blood chemistry. It is also the test that the clinician faces in the diagnostic evaluation of a patient.

Hematology is the specialty of medicine that studies the blood and the hematopoietic tissues that comprise it, such as: bone marrow, spleen, lymph nodes, and all structural and biochemical hematological disorders that lead to disease.

Blood cytometry describes the laboratory study in this area that is intended to provide information on the number and characteristics of blood cells such as their size, shape and volume (6).

In this area we count blood cells through spectrophotometry, identify cells through staining and study the time it takes to form a clot in the organism. All this is done through automated equipment in order to deliver results that are as accurate as possible.

Therefore, the correct clinical interpretation of blood cytometry values the analysis that is considered a test that yields three major groups: each with different functions, but sharing a common origin in the bone marrow: data from the red series, the white series, and the thrombocyte series. (7)

The measurement of all parameters and indices is done using particle counters by means of flow cytometry through the "Coulter" equipment, so the results obtained are necessary to establish the reference values.

The reference values of cytometry in general are variable and depend on different factors, such as: age, sex, height of place of residence, among others. These parameters are variable in each laboratory (8).

10.1 Red Series

The data reported by blood cytometry for the red series are as follows:

10.1.1 Hemoglobin (Hb)

Hemoglobin is the globular protein contained in large quantities in the erythrocyte, it contains iron, and its main function is to transport oxygen from the pulmonary alveoli and carry it to the tissues, and in turn to collect the CO_2 produced and carry it back to the lungs, to be released and retake the O_2. The CO_2 that is not transported by Hb will be dissolved in the plasma in the form of bicarbonate. It is also the protein responsible for giving the blood its red color (9).

Hemoglobin is measured in grams per deciliter (g/dL) and represents the amount of hemoglobin per unit volume. This parameter should be the only one to be used to define whether or not there is anemia, i.e., if the hemoglobin figures are below normal values, anemia may be present.

Healthy adults range from 12.5-16.6 g/dL for women and 15.5-19.5 g/dL for men. Figures lower than 12.5 for women and 15.5 for men allow the diagnosis of anemia to be established. And hemoglobin figures higher than 16.6 g/dl for women and 19.5 g/dl for men allow establishing the diagnosis of erythrocytosis. (6)

10.1.2 Hematocrit (Hct)

It is measured as a percentage and represents the volume of the erythrocyte portion in relation to the total blood volume. The reference hematocrit ranges from 39 to 50% for women and 46 to 56% for men. This parameter is calculated from the measurement of the number of erythrocytes and mean globular volume, therefore, it is a parameter with lower precision than the other two. Its number depends on the size of the red blood cell (6).

It is a parameter that with a single data, the clinician gets an overall idea of the patient's blood status, but taking into account the state of hydration, as dehydration increases it considerably.

Decreased hematocrit may indicate anemia, blood loss, red blood cell destruction, leukemia, nutritional deficiencies and overhydration.

A high value translates into polycythemia, congenital heart disease, lung tumors, cancer, dehydration, erythrocytosis, low oxygen levels, polycythemia vera or fibrosis.

10.1.3 Red blood cell count (RBC)

The red blood cells carry oxygen to the lungs to the rest of the body. And it also carries carbon dioxide back to the lungs so that it can be exhaled.

Red blood cell count is measured in millions per microliter (millions/µl). The reference values in adults are women 4.1 to 5.7 million/µl and men 5.0 to 6.3 million/µl. (6)

If the red blood cell count is low it is known as anemia, and if it is too high it would be a disease called polycythemia.

10.1.4 Mean globular volume (MGV)

Represents the measurement of erythrocyte size. It is measured in femtoliters (fL) or cubic microns. This erythrocyte index is of great value in clarifying the cause of anemia. The values of the eGV allow to know if an anemia is macrositic (eGV increased to normal limits) or micrositic (eGV decreased to normal limits) ranging from 78 to 103 fL for women and 83 to 98 fL for men.

10.1.5 Mean corpuscular hemoglobin (MCH)

It is expressed in picograms (pg) and represents the average amount of hemoglobin in each erythrocyte. The parameters for MCH are from 27 to 34 pg in each erythrocyte, i.e., it is used to refer to the amount of hemoglobin contained; we will speak of hypochromia and normochromia when the value of MCH is subnormal or normal, respectively. (6)

This parameter indicates the average amount of hemoglobin contained in each hematie or red blood cell. Thanks to this parameter it is possible to classify anemias in a different way: hypochromias are those with a low level of MCH and hyperchromias are those with a high level of MCH.

10.1.6 Hemoglobin concentration

Hemoglobin concentration is a directly measured parameter. After the counting cycles are completed, the leukocyte dilution is passed to the hemoglobinometer for hemoglobin determination. Lithium reagent is added to the dilution to lyse or break up the erythrocytes and convert the released hemoglobin into a stable cyanide pigment that can be measured photometrically. The more hemoglobin present in the sample, the more light is absorbed.

10.1.7 Mean globular hemoglobin concentration (CmHb)

This erythrocyte index, measured as a percentage (%), refers to the measure of hemoglobin concentration in a given volume of red blood cells.

The reference values of CmHb are 30 to 34% for women and 32 to 34% for men. If the index exceeds the established values, it is referred to as absolute hyperchromia.

10.1.8 Coefficient of variation of VGM (CV-VGM)

It is measured as a percentage (%) where it is calculated with the flow cytometer by means of frequency distribution histograms of erythrocyte volumes. This index is also known as "red cell distribution width" (RDW). The flow cytometry equipment makes an erythrocyte size distribution curve (ESV), where it plots on the abscissa the ESV measured in femtoliters and on the ordinates the relative frequency of the volumes, expressed in (%). The CV-VGM is approximately 12 to 13% under normal conditions.

10.1.9 Erythrocyte count

In the automated system the erythrocyte count is a directly measured parameter. The dilution contains erythrocytes, leukocytes and platelets. Particles that are 36 fL or larger are counted as erythrocytes. The leukocytes present in the dilution are included in the erythrocyte count, their interference is usually negligible because they are only a few thousand compared to the millions of erythrocytes. The erythrocyte mean corpuscular volume (MCV) is its average taken from the size distribution data. Hematocrit (Hto), mean corpuscular hemoglobin (MCH) and mean corpuscular hemoglobin concentration (MCHC) are calculated from measured and derived values. The amplitude of the erythrocyte distribution is calculated directly from the histogram as the coefficient of variation (CV) of the erythrocyte volume distribution.

10.1.10 Reticulocyte count

Reticulocytes are larger than hematocytes and have a fine granulofilamentous network in their cytoplasm corresponding to altered ribosomal RNA remnants. Their normal numbers are 0.5 to 1.5/100 hematies and in absolute number 25,000 to 75,000 per $mm3$.

Reticulocyte counts are fundamental in the study of anemia. It allows us to know the medullary reactive capacity and to orient the origin of the anemia towards an extramedullary mechanism if there is reticulocytosis which demonstrates a good response capacity of the bone marrow (regenerative anemias) and in the opposite direction if there is reticulocytopenia it leads us to classify the anemia as hyporenerative due to structural or functional failure of the bone marrow.

They reflect the production of erythrocytes by the bone marrow. They are immature cells that circulate in the blood for 48 h before becoming mature erythrocytes. A normal result for healthy adults is about 0.5 to 1.5%.

Analyzers evaluate reticulocytes by optical scattering, after treating the erythrocytes with nucleic acid dyes, which is indicated by the existence of residual RNA that precipitates with certain dyes, such as methylene blue, then a portion of the collected blood is washed to remove the hemoglobin but preserve the RNA in the cell. This portion of the sample is aspirated into the flow cell and the cells are measured. The flow cell analyzes approximately 10,000 cells to determine the percentage of reticulocytes as well as their absolute number. This is an indirect indication of the extent of erythropoiesis in the bone marrow.

10.1.11 Interpretation of the results obtained from the red series

In summary, all low or high values of the above mentioned parameters go hand in hand, a good interpretation by the physician is essential to arrive at a diagnosis. Some of the interpretations of the parameters are described here.

<u>Low levels result in:</u>

- Reduced red blood cell production in the bone marrow

- Anemia of various types

- Renal diseases

- Deficient nutrition (iron, folate, B12 or B6)

- Autoimmune diseases

- Cancer

- Hemorrhages

<u>A high level translates into:</u>

- Abnormal increase in bone marrow red blood cell production to compensate for low oxygen levels.

- Congenital heart disease, heart failure

- Chronic lung diseases

- Smoking

- Dehydration

- Taking hormones for sports enhancement such as erythropoietin.

- Polycythemia.

- Living at high altitude

10.2 White series

Known as white blood cells because they lack pigment, they can be observed macroscopically in a resting blood sample and are found in clusters exhibiting a creamy whitish color. Their initial assessment consists of the total quantitative interpretation of the cellular subtypes.

leukocytes are cells, which unlike erythrocytes, do have a nucleus and a series of cytoplasmic organelles that are spherical in shape and are usually modified into amoeboid or pleomorphic forms when they leave the bloodstream and perform their functions in the interstitial tissue of the circulating blood, which allows them to be easily differentiated from the other cells present. Leukocytes do not function within the bloodstream, but travel from one region of the body to another, having the ability to leave the blood capillaries by movements (diapedesis) and thus reach the tissues where they exert their action. Leukocytes are attracted to the tissues by a series of chemical or viral substances that produce infection or by substances released by the activated cells and tissues.

Leukocytes derive from the bone marrow, originate from the myeloid stem cell (granulocytes and monocytes) and others from the lymphoid stem cell (lymphocytes), some of them, such as lymphocytes, acquire their functional capacity in the parenchyma of the spleen, thymus, lymph nodes, tonsils and lymph follicles located in the digestive, respiratory and urogenital apparatus. They have a half-life of a few hours ranging from 9 to 10 days approximately (10).

10.2.1 Number of white blood cells (WBC)

The variation of the leukocyte count helps the physician to diagnose some diseases on the basis of their increase or decrease. Their main function is to participate in the body's defense against infections, and the number may increase in acute rheumatic fever, acidosis, acute gout, poisoning, acute hemorrhage, acute leukemia, polycythemia vera, tension, menstruation, gangrene, infarction, appendicitis, pneumonia, abscesses, and this increase is known as leukocytosis. They can also decrease in number in bacterial infections such as septicemia, miliary tuberculosis, typhoid, brucellosis; viral infections such as hepatitis, influenza, mumps, other infections such as malaria, and some medications such as antibiotics, analgesics, myelosuppressive antithyroid drugs, ionizing radiation, pernicious anemia, bone marrow aplasia, generalized lupus erythematosus, rheumatoid arthritis, renal failure, cancer, and this state is known as leukopenia.

The number of leukocytes is measured in billions per liter ($x10^9$ /L). The number also depends on many factors such as age, weight, smoking habits, use of contraceptive hormones, etc. For adults the reference values range between 4 and 12 x 10^9 /L (4000 to 12 000 /µL). (6)

10.2.2 Differential white blood cell count

It consists of a white blood cell count, and in blood cytometry is of fundamental character, the cell count is expressed as a percentage and consists of the leukocyte count. A correct interpretation by the physician allows the identification of infectious and inflammatory diseases, leukemia, lymphoma and bone marrow disorders.

The following types of leukocytes can be found in peripheral blood: neutrophils or polymorphonuclears (including segmented nuclei, banded nuclei and metamyelocytes), eosinophils, basophils, lymphocytes and monocytes (11).

They are classified into two groups:

- Granulocytes, which have specific glands in their cytoplasm.

- Agranulocytes, which lack specific granules.

There are three types of granulocytes, which differ according to the color of their specific granules.

- Neutrophils

- Eosinophils

- Basophils

There are two types of Agranulocytes.

- Lymphocytes

- Monocytes

Due to the large volume of tests performed in the laboratory and the amount of work, doing it manually would be very heavy and slow, today we opt for the use of technology, creating automatic counters that perform this function, since currently this function is performed automatically in all laboratories, leaving manual counting in the background. In adults, the normal ratio is shown in the table below.

Cell	Percentage (%)	Absolute limits (μl).
Total neutrophils	40-85	1 500-7 000
Metamyelocytes	0-2	<10-500
In band	0-11	100-800
Segmented	40-74	2 000-6 00
Eosinophils	0-7	<100-200
Basophils	<10-20	<10-20
Monocytes	1-13	100-800
Lymphocytes	12-46	1 000-4 200

Figure 7. Differential leukocyte count.

10.2.3 Leukocyte count

This parameter is measured directly by the Coulter analyzer, and to generate blood biometry data including leukocyte count, in a separate channel to evaluate the leukocyte differential determination in five components.

Classification according to cell volumetric size is allowed by impedance, cell conductivity measurements and laser light scattering all performed simultaneously for each cell.

Particles between 35 and 90 fL are considered lymphocytes, between 90 and 160 fL, "mononuclear" (monocytes, blasts, immature granulocytes and lymphocytes), and between 160 and 450 fL granulocytes, thus making it possible to calculate the relative and absolute numbers of these populations.

After lysing the erythrocytes and treating the leukocytes with a stabilizing reagent to maintain them in a "near native" state, a focused sample current is directed through the cell flow path through the sensing zone. The low-frequency DC current measures size while a high-frequency electromagnetic probe measures conductivity; an indicator of internal cellular content. Each cell is also analyzed with monochromatic laser light that reveals information about the cell surface such as its structure, shape and reflectivity, which is the ability to reflect a certain amount of light. More than 8,000 leukocytes are analyzed in each sample.

Three direct measurements (volume, conductivity and light scattering) are taken for each leukocyte as it passes through the opening of a flow cell. These data are recorded three-dimensionally, cell populations are identified and percentages are reported.

10.2.4 Neutrophils

They are the most abundant cells, under normal conditions, they exist in a percentage of 60-70% of the total leukocytes, in absolute numbers they are considered from 3000 to 6000 per μl.

Their cytoplasm has specific granules, which are very small and abundant (containing bacteriostatic agents), stained violet with a mixture of acidic (eosin) and basic (methylene blue) dyes, and nonspecific or azurophilic granules, which are larger and less numerous (containing myeloperoxidase, lysosomal enzymes and defensins).

Their nuclei are lobulated and are joined by thin chromatic bridges forming 3 to 6 lobules; the number of lobules depends on the age of the cell.

Neutrophils are one of the first cells to appear in acute bacterial infection and are important in the inflammatory reaction of the organism, they are involved in active phagocytosis of bacteria, foreign microorganisms, passive phagocytosis of connective tissue cells, damaged erythrocytes and fibrin.

When the neutrophil phagocytes and digests a bacterium or microorganism, some perish in the process, and constitute an accumulation of dead bacteria and neutrophils forming the yellowish exudate called pus.

Cytometry determines the presence of neutrophilia, which is the increase in the absolute number of neutrophils in response to invading microorganisms or neoplastic cells. Neutropenia occurs when too few neutrophils are produced in the bone marrow and too many are stored in the margins of the blood vessels (12).

10.2.5 Eosinophils

They constitute less than 4% of the total white blood cell population, in absolute numbers considered normal 150-450 mm^3 of blood, tend to be slightly larger than neutrophils, contain a bilobed nucleus, two lobules separated or joined by a small chromatin can. The cytoplasm contains specific granules of an intense pink or red color (stained with eosin) and few azurophilic granules.

The granules exert an intense cytotoxic effect on protozoa and parasitic helminths, they are able to digest the wall of metazoa, generating substances capable of regulating the inflammatory process, as well as intervening in allergic disorders.

The cytoplasm contains in its interior structures in the form of crystals called internum effective in the destruction of parasites and also has neurotoxins, also involved in the fight against infections, makes its appearance after the acute phase occurs, is responsible for cleaning the cells of bacteria and dead neutrophils, and is believed to combat the effects of histamine and other mediators of inflammation (12).

The number of eosinophils increases in processes in which there is parasitic infection or allergic reactions. They are abundant in the nasal secretion and in the sputum of those suffering from asthma due to allergy.

10.2.6 Basophils

They are the least numerous leukocytes, constituting 0.5 to 1% of the total white blood cells.

The basophil nucleus is also lobulated, it can be trilobed or s-shaped, half of the cell is constituted by the nucleus which usually has 2 to 3 lobes connected by chromatin bridges and can be segmented and regular in shape. In most cases the outline of the nucleus is not easily seen, because it is hidden by the specific granules which are stained dark blue (stained with methylene blue).

Its granules contain heparin which is an anticoagulant and histamine, a vasodilator substance that dilates small vessels, constituting 50% of the histamine present in blood, thus acting as a chemotactic factor of eosinophils, and peroxidase, so it is thought to participate in allergic reactions, In plasma it has receptors for immunoglobulin IgE, when IgE binds to the receptor, the cell is activated and the granulation cell is initiated, which releases vasoactive enzymes, bronchoconstrictors and chemoattractants (especially for neutrophils).

Basophil functions as a mediator of inflammatory responses such as hypersensitivity, is associated with anaphylactic reactions, myelo-proliferative diseases, and immunity against parasites and allergies (12).

10.2.7 Lymphocytes

They are small cells, and constitute 20% to 30% of the total white blood cells.

They have a voluminous spherical nucleus that occupies almost all the cytoplasm and is situated around the nucleus in the form of a ring. This cytoplasm exhibits a slight basophilia. Some lymphocytes present nuclei with a slight cleavage in which the cytoplasm has few azurophilic globules (nonspecific granulation), there are three types of lymphocytes: B, T and null cells or NK lymphocytes.

Lymphocytes are not functional within the bloodstream, they develop in the bone marrow and also in tissues called primary and secondary lymphoid organs, the primary organs being the thymus and bone marrow, while the secondary organs are the spleen, Peyer's patches, tonsils and lymph nodes distributed throughout the body. They acquire immunological capacity when they go to the bone marrow to differentiate into B lymphocytes and when they go to the cortex of the thymus to transform into T lymphocytes.

The main function of the lymphocyte is the regulation of immune function as it plays a fundamental role in immune relations. If a foreign material (exogenous antigenic material, dead or malignant cells) is completely engulfed, it is degraded and eliminated by the action of phagocytes and no immune response is produced, and if complete engulfment does not occur, a series of reactions, factors, biochemical and morphological events are triggered that stimulate lymphocyte activation.

T lymphocytes participate in the cell-mediated immune response, and exist in 15% of the percentage of total lymphocytes, B cells participate in the production, synthesis and secretion of antibodies making up 80%, and NK cells can destroy foreign cells, cancerous or altered by viruses without the need for medication of cooperating lymphocytes, making up the other 5%. (12)

10.2.8 Monocytes

They constitute only 3 to 8% of the leukocytes in normal blood, are the largest white blood cells observed in a smear, their nucleus is bulky and occupies half of the cell, is usually located in an extrinsic position and adopts an irregular shape, commonly described as horseshoe cell, or rounded shape.

When the foreign body is of considerable size, several monocytes fuse and form multinucleated giant cells, termed "foreign body giant cells". More than 50 secretory compounds, such as transport proteins, nonspecific inflammatory agents, depot materials and humoral agents, are identified in monocytes.

Monocytes also penetrate connective tissue during inflammation and transform into macrophages that phagocytize cells and tissue debris, fibrin, remnant bacteria and can destroy tumor cells.

Macrophages: the macrophage eventually leaves the blood and enters the tissues where it matures into a macrophage. The transformation from monocyte to macrophage is characterized by progressive growth. The nucleus becomes round, nucleoli appear and the cytoplasm appears blue in color, in addition to showing a large number of granules. The monocyte-macrophage or mononuclear phagocytic system plays an important role in the initiation and regulation of the immune response (12).

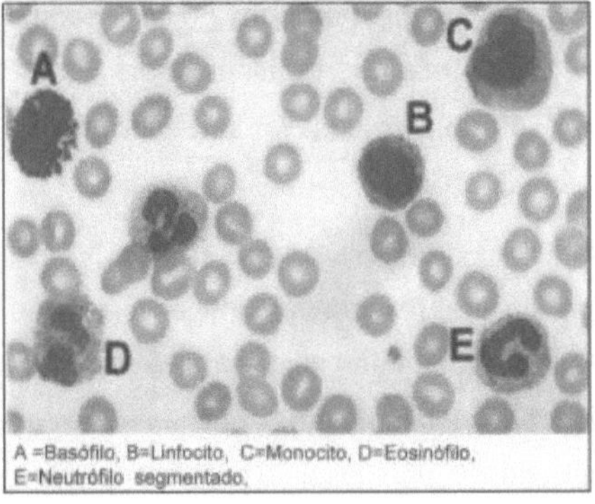

Figure 8. Five types of leukocytes.

10.3 Thrombotic series

Platelets or thrombocytes are the smallest elements, very tiny, approximately 1 to 4 µm in diameter. Like the other blood cells, they are also formed in the bone marrow from megakaryocytes, which are very large cells that, when fragmented (in the bone marrow, on entering the peripheral blood or by compression by the capillaries) form the tiny platelets, which is why they contain no nucleus, i.e. they are not true cells but cytoplasmic fragments. The fundamental task of platelets is the activation of blood coagulation, playing a fundamental role in the process of hemostasis. When observed under the microscope, using Wright's stain we can see how their center is intensely tinged (13).

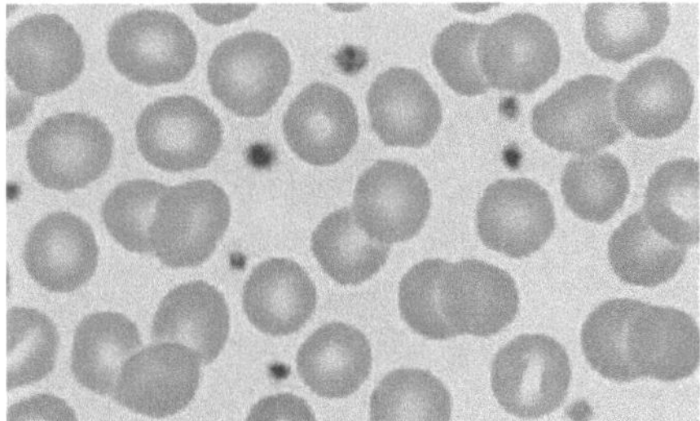

Figure 9. Platelets are stained more intensely and are characterized by their small size.

10.3.1 Platelet count (PLT)

The reference platelet count is between 150 and 500 $\times 10^9$ /L (150 000 to 500 000/µl). A lower number in the blood circulation is called thrombocytopenia and an excess of platelets is called thrombositosis.

The causes of thrombocytopenia are: autoimmune purpura, acute leukemia, aplastic anemia, pernicious anemia, blood transfusions, lupus, etc. When the platelet count is above 500 000/µl, we speak of thrombosis, whose causes are also multiple: malignant diseases, myeloproliferative syndromes such as polycythemia vera, chronic myeloid leukemia, primary thrombosis, etc. (6).

10.3.2 Platelet count

Although platelets are measured directly, channels are used for platelet analysis. Platelets are counted within the limits of 2 to 20 fL and a size distribution histogram is constructed. In general, platelet size is inversely proportional to platelet count.

10.3.3 Parameters for platelets

Mean Platelet Volume (MPV). It is a parameter that measures the size of platelets in the blood, the unit of measurement is in femtoliters (fL) and its normal value is 7.5 to 10 fL. MPV measures platelet volume, which is directly related to platelet size. In thrombocytopenia the volume is elevated and in thrombositosis it is decreased, thus, there is an inverse relationship between the number of platelets and MPV (14).

Platelet volume distribution (PDW). It indicates the degree of uniformity in platelet size, measuring whether there are large differences in platelet size from one platelet to another, assisting in the identification of serious platelet abnormalities.

10.4 Manual methods in the laboratory

10.4.1 Blood smear

The practice of the blood smear, also called extended smear, is of great importance in hematology since the diagnosis of many hematological diseases can be made by simply observing the morphological characteristics of the blood cells, so it should not be too thick or too thin.

After the sample is taken, and before disposing of the syringe to the RPBIs, a small drop of blood is placed on the base of a slide, in order to perform a peripheral blood smear, by applying a staining method that facilitates the microscopic observation of the cells that make up the blood. All this in order to observe the white blood cells and make a count expressed as a percentage called differential blood cell banks. There is a machine with a recorder that contains keys for the different types of cells, the keys will be recorded and will alert when 100 cells have been counted. After a microscopic count, the percentages of each sample are determined and then compared with the normal percentages.

All films to be used for the smear, especially new ones, should be cleaned with absorbent cotton and 70% alcohol to remove adhering grease.

For a smear to be of good quality it must cover 80% of the laminin with head, body and tail. Thick smears make it difficult to visualize and identify cells, while thin smears result in an abnormal distribution of the leukocyte elements present. Before starting the staining, the laminin is examined to check if the cellular elements are well distributed (15).

10.4.2 Two-slide method

On one slide place another slide on the surface of the first slide (on which the drop of blood is located) forming an angle of 45°, slide gently and at moderate speed the slide over the other slide lengthwise until the drop of blood is well spread on the surface of the first slide. The thickness of the blood smear can vary according to the angle between the two slides. Thus, if it is greater than 45°, the smear obtained will be thick and short, if it is less than 45° it will be long and thin. The smear is dried at room temperature and in horizontal position.

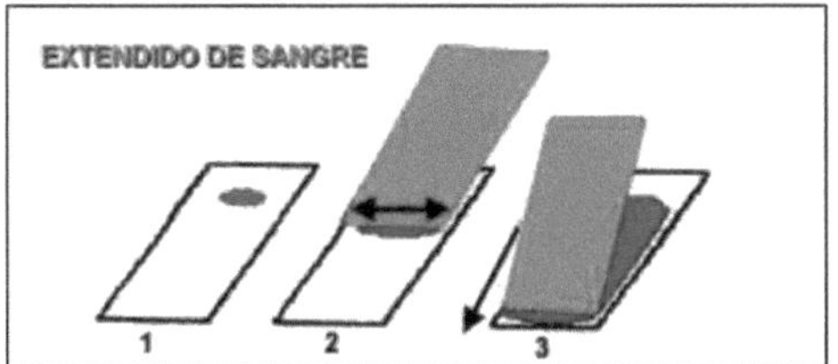

Figure 10. Spread on peripheral blood slides.

10.4.3 Staining with Wright's dye

Wright's stain will provide a means to study the blood and determine variations and abnormalities in erythrocyte structure, shape and size, hemoglobin content and staining properties. The information obtained from a peripheral blood smear depends largely on the quality of the smear and the staining.

Once the blood smear is obtained, it is left to dry for 15 to 20 min, then the slide is covered with Wright's dye for 5 minutes, then a buffered solution is added until a metallic shine is obtained, leaving an additional 5 minutes, and finally it is washed with running water and left to dry. The slide is placed in the microscope adding a drop of immersion oil, focused at a magnification of 100x and, at low magnification, the quality of the staining is checked, the approximate number of white blood cells and the site is chosen to start the count.

This makes it possible to differentiate five types of leukocytes that can be classified by two criteria:

a)   Core shape.

b)   Presence or absence of specific granules.

When blood cells are suspended in blood plasma and spread on slides (blood smears), the granules differ in color when a mixed or neutral stain is applied, consisting of acid and base colors, depending on the procedure, e.g., eosin (acid stain) and methylene blue (base stain).

According to the shape of the nucleus and the presence or absence of granules, the eukocytes are named:

1.   Polymorphous nuclear or granulocytes. They have lobulated nuclei and possess, in the cytoplasm, specific granules that are selectively stained with a certain color, e.g.

neutrophils, eosinophils and basophils.

2. Mononuclear or agranulocytes. They have spherical or slightly scolexed nuclei, without lobulations; the cytoplasm lacks specific granulations, examples: lymphocytes and normocytes.

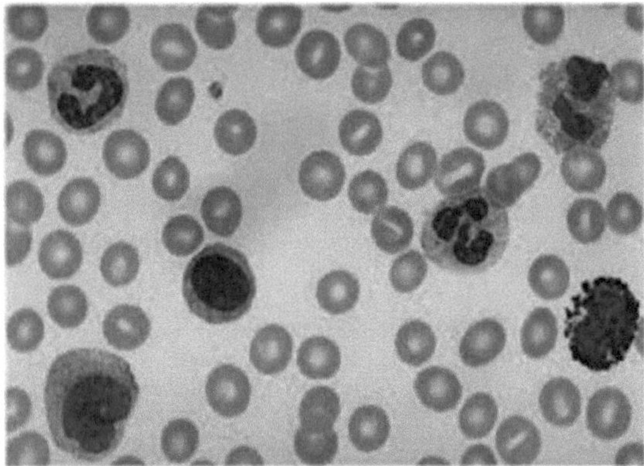

Figure 11. Cells stained with Wright's stain.

10.5 Automated Flow Cytometer Method

The measurement of all parameters in the laboratory is done using flow cytometry particle counters, there is an extensive line of blood analyzers, equipment that provides a complete analysis of erythrocytes, platelets and leukocytes with differential counting of five components and fully automated online reticulocyte analysis. The flow cytometer is a computer-aided instrument that determines the physical characteristics of each cell with a laser light source.

Flow cytometry is a multiparametric cell analysis technique based on passing a suspension of particles (usually cells) aligned one by one in front of a focused laser beam. The impact of each cell with the light beam produces signals corresponding to different parameters of the cell, which are picked up by different detectors. The detectors convert these signals into electronic signals that are then digitized to allow the simultaneous measurement of several parameters in the same cell, these are parameters related to intrinsic characteristics of the cell, such as its size and the complexity of the nucleus and cytoplasm. Flow cytometry is therefore able to identify a cell by its morphological characteristics of size and complexity.

The measurement of each of the parameters that make up blood biometry is performed on a Coulter instrument, which is an automated hematological analyzer for in vitro diagnostic use in the clinical laboratory. Coulter is a flow cytometer using VCS (Volume, Conductivity and Scatter) technology that allows cell sorting according to volumetric size and physical characteristics with a laser light source performed simultaneously.

A laser is a hollow, closed tube containing an inert gas, such as argon, helium or neon. Passing an electric current through this gas-filled tube produces an intense laser light called monochromatic, since it is emitted as a single wavelength, which excites the inert gas molecules at a higher energy level. When these excited ions return to their natural state of low entropy, the energy is released in the form of a photon of light. The light in the laser tube is intensified by a series of mirrors and finally emitted as a narrow beam of light of a single specific wavelength. The wavelength of the monochromatic light is characteristic of the gas inside the laser tube.

A sample is aspirated into the tubing containing a stream of liquid moving towards the periphery (the shell) and a central stream of liquid (the sample with the cells). The sample stream is hydrodynamically centered on a single line of particles or cells by adjusting the external pressure on the jacket and the velocity of the stream. This causes the cells to move in a single row in front of the laser beam, like beads on a string in the center of the liquid stream. The term used for the movement of two liquids passing each other without mixing is laminar flow. The laser beam is focused on individual cells by a series of lenses and prisms. This light can be measured as it is reflected or scattered away from the cells. Two basic principles are used to operate this equipment: electronic impedance and optical scattering.

•   Electronic impedance. The principle of impedance in blood cell counting is based on the increase in resistance produced when a blood cell with low conductivity passes through an electric field. The number of flashes indicates the number of blood cells, and the amplitude of each flash is proportional to the volume of the cell.

•   Optical scattering. The principle of optical light scattering in blood cell counting is based on light scattering measurements obtained from a single blood cell passing through a light beam (laser). The blood cells create a forward and a side scatter which are detected by photodetectors.

The blood analyzer has some basic components such as: the hydraulic, pneumatic and electrical system.

The hydraulic system includes the suction unit, dispensers, diluents, mixing chambers, opening baths, cell flow or both, and a hemoglobinometer.

The pneumatic system includes the vacuum and pressures required to operate the valves and transport the sample through the hydraulic system.

The electrical system controls the operational sequences of the total system and includes electronic analyzers and computerized circuits for processing the data generated.

The Coulter equipment has two measurement channels in the hydraulic system to determine hematological biometry data: erythrocyte and leukocyte counts, and hemoglobin determination (HGB) are measured directly.

The samples are placed in a rack with the barcode on the front, so that the sample can be identified by the equipment's barcode reader and analyzed.

The whole blood sample (EDTA anticoagulated) aspirate is divided into two portions and each portion is mixed with an isotonic diluent. The first dilution is delivered to the erythrocyte opening chamber and the second to the leukocyte opening chamber.

In the first case, erythrocytes and platelets are counted and differentiated by electrical impedance as the cells pass through each of the three sensor apertures (50µ diameter, 60µ length). Particles between 2 and 20 femtoliters (fL) are counted as platelets and those over 36 fL are counted as erythrocytes. In the leukocyte chamber, a reagent is added to lyse the erythrocytes and release the hemoglobin before counting the leukocytes simultaneously by impedance in each of the three sensing apertures (100µ diameter, 75µ length).

The electrical pulses generated in the counting cycles are sent to the analyzer for review, match correction and digital conversion. Two of the three counts obtained in the erythrocyte and leukocyte containers must agree. (12)

1.1.11 Sample processing

The sample processing by the Coulter requires purple tubes containing EDTA that prevent the sample from coagulating, another very important fact is that the equipment homogenizes the sample very well before starting the cell counting process, in addition to the process that is done for the use of the equipment is narrated in the following steps:

1.   Enter in the equipment the mandatory data suggested by the equipment, such as: the folio number of the sample, year, month and day of birth, full name, sex, physician requesting the study, and add the number of the tube holder where the sample will be placed.

2.   Save the results in the equipment and proceed to give the order to start processing

the sample.

Once the operation has been completed by the team after its analysis, all the results obtained, including the histogram, are reviewed. If required, the results are printed on letterhead.

10.6 Erythrocyte sedimentation rate

The erythrocyte sedimentation rate (ESR) is useful to monitor the evolution of an inflammatory disease or to differentiate similar diseases, it is a test that is always requested by the physician together with other tests, in order to detect inflammation associated with infections, cancers and diseases.

The erythrocyte sedimentation rate is elevated in patients presenting with rheumatic fever, rheumatoid arthritis or pyogenic arthritis. It is elevated in the early stages of acute pelvic inflammatory disease or ruptured ectopic pregnancy, but is normal in the first 24 hours of acute appendicitis. It can be used to indicate active pulmonary tuberculosis. In addition, this test is also requested to monitor the activity and response of the organism to treatment based on a disease process. Such may be the case with systemic lupus erythematosus.

It is quite unspecific because it does not tell the doctor the exact place in the body where an inflammation is located, nor does it say much about the origin of the cause, which is why it is requested along with more laboratory tests.

The principle of sedimentation occurs when anticoagulated blood is left to stand for a period of time at room temperature, the erythrocytes settle to the bottom of the tube due to gravity. The ESR is the number of millimeters that erythrocytes sediment in 1 hour, which is affected by erythrocyte, plasma, mechanical and technical factors. Erythrocytes have a net negative surface charge, therefore they tend to repel each other; the repulsive forces are partially or totally neutralized if there is an increase in the amount of positively charged plasma proteins; erythrocytes sediment faster due to the formation of erythrocyte aggregates or "rollers". Some diseases, such as multiple myeloma, can cause the formation of rollers due to altered fibrinogen and plasma globulins. Normal erythrocytes have a relatively small mass, and sediment slowly. (15)

ESR is usually determined using the Wintrobe tube by the following procedure.

1.   Obtain the blood sample placed in Vacutainer tubes containing EDTA as anticoagulant previously homogenized.

2.   Fill the Wintrobe pipette up to the zero millimeter mark making sure that there should

be no air bubbles in the pipette.

3.   Place the pipette in the holder in a vertical position, at a 90° angle.

4.   Set the timer for one hour and allow to settle without touching for 60 minutes.

5.   After 60 minutes read the number of milliliters that the erythrocytes descended, the leukocyte layer should not be included in the reading. ESR is reported as mm/h.

The reference values are: Women up to 20mm/h and Men up to 15mm/h.

The causes of elevated values with increased sedimentation are: pregnancy, aging, severe anemia, chronic inflammatory process, acute myocardial infarction, renal failure, neoplasms, hemopathies and tumors. Causes of decreased values with lower sedimentation are: polycythemia, erythrocyte alteration, etc.

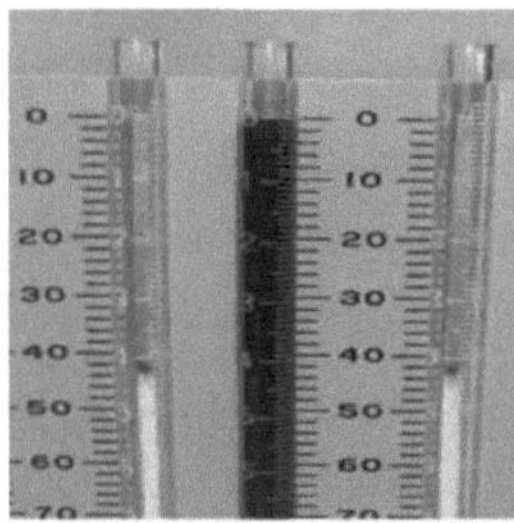

Figure 12. ESR in Wintrobe tube.

10.7 Blood group

The blood group of each individual is determined by a series of antigens present in their blood cells, leukocytes, platelets, and even in their serum. The antigens on which we are going to base ourselves will be the erythrocytic ones because they are the best known.

At present, more than 400 different erythrocyte antigens are known (most of them are glycolipids and mocopolysaccharides), which will join together to form different systems. Given the number of possible combinations, we can say that the blood group of each individual is practically unrepeatable, and therefore personal.

Blood antigens are inherited according to Mendel's laws, presenting paternal and maternal antigens that will determine their blood group, the individual will have the same blood group throughout life, there are several systems in which you can gather all these different antigens: the best known is ABO and Rh System discovered by Landsteiner in 1901 is based on 2 glucogenic antigens naturally present in erythrocytes; in this way we can have the following 4 ABO groups: (16)

*   Group A, which presents antigen A

*   Group B, which presents antigen B

*   Group AB presenting both A and B antigens.

*   Group O, which does not present any type of antigen.

In addition, these groups present an agglutinin that would attack the antigen not present in their blood, so that the antigen would not be present in their blood:

*   Group A, has anti-B agglutinin present.

*   Group B has agglutinin A present.

*   Group AB, has no agglutinin present because it has both antigens in its blood.

*   Group O, has both agglutinins present because it does not have any antigen in its blood.

Logically, no group will have an agglutinin against its own antigen.

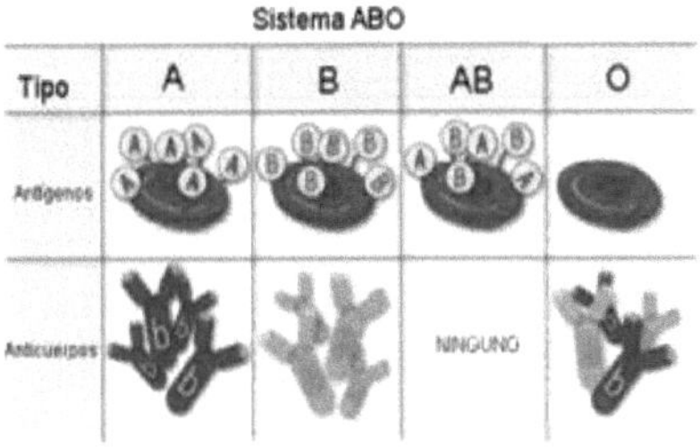

Figure 13. ABO system.

The Rh system discovered by Landsteiner and Wiener in 1940 is the second most important due to the post-transfusion hemolytic reactions it triggers and, above all, due to the feto-maternal incompatibility for which it is responsible. As in the ABO system, antigens appear in the blood that will determine whether the individual is Rh (positive) or Rh (negative).

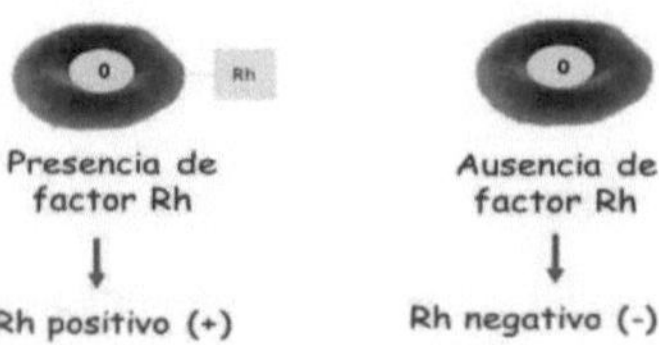

Figure 14. Rh positive and negative system.

The test for blood grouping and Rh can be performed immediately by obtaining blood directly from the finger with an aseptic lancet prick. The puncture should be made sharply and deep enough for the blood to flow freely from the finger. There is no need to apply pressure, but blood can also be preserved with EDTA for 48 hours refrigerated at 2-8 °C. To avoid errors, two controls, a positive and a negative control, should be placed next to the Rh.

The test is performed on a slide as follows:

1.   Three 30 µL drops of blood are placed on a slide with the aid of the micropipette, one on the right, one in the center and one on the left.

2.   To the first drop of blood is added 30 µL of anti-A reagent, to the second drop of blood is added 30 µL anti-B reagent and to the third drop of blood is added 30 µL of anti-D reagent.

3.   The blood and the reagent are mixed well with the help of a wooden stick, discarding the wooden stick in the trash for each mixture.

4.   It is subjected to pendulum movements for two minutes to observe the presence of agglutination.

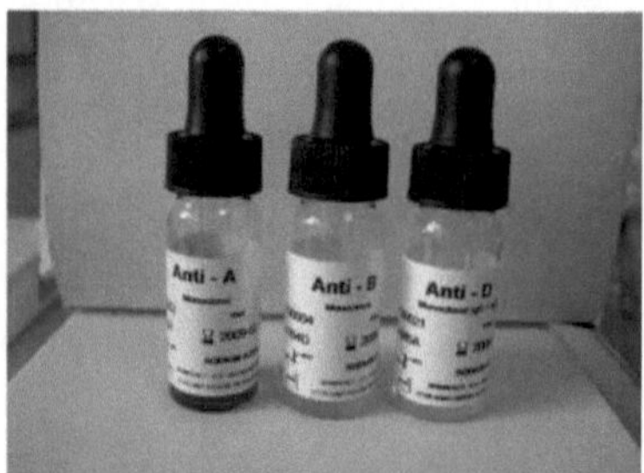

Figure 15. Reagents for blood group determination.

Negative reaction: no visible sign of agglutination, this negativity must be confirmed.

Positive reaction: visible agglutination.

The reactions obtained on the slide are due to the fact that in the cellular plasma of each person there are antibodies, produced by the B lymphocyte, against the antigens not present in their hematopoiesis. Thus the individual belonging to group A has anti-B antibodies, while the one belonging to group B has anti-A antibodies, the one belonging to group O has neither antigen A nor B, and the one belonging to group AB has both antigens, and therefore does not have antibodies against them.

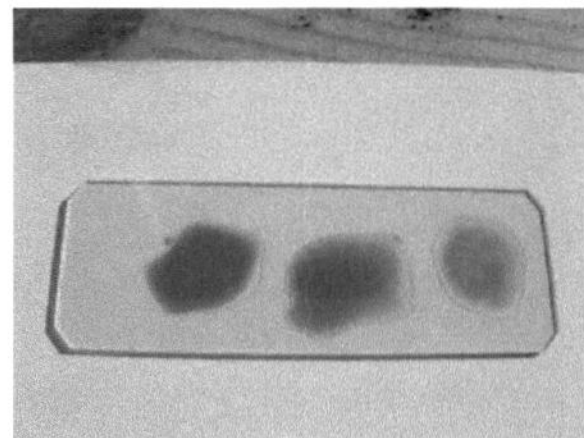

Figure 18. Type O blood (-)

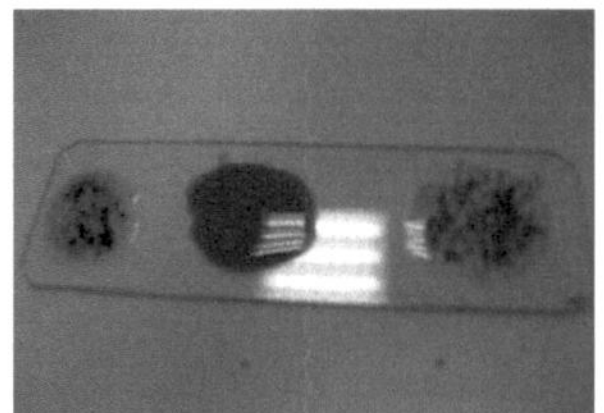

Figure 19. Blood type A (+)

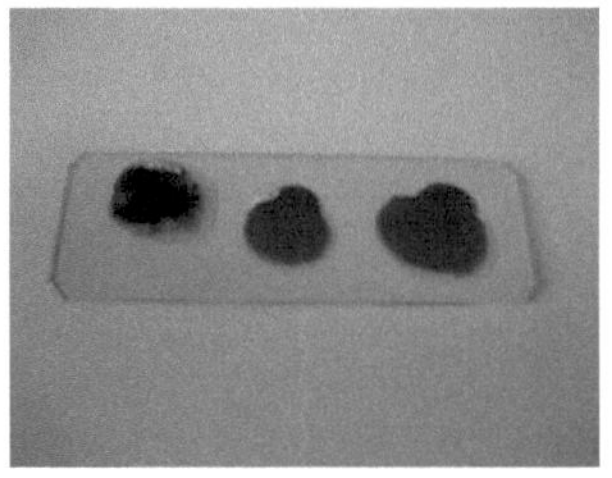

Figure 17. Blood type A (-)

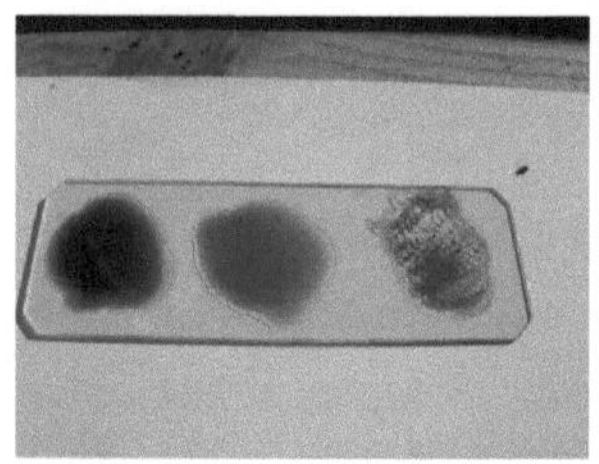

Figure 16. Blood type O (+)

10.8 Coagulation

In the coagulation area different routine and useful tests are processed for the diagnosis and control of bleeding disorders, thrombosis and hypercoagulability states, by means of tests that guide a clinical diagnosis. Here are quantified coagulation factors and proteins involved in this process, all in an automated way.

The prothrombin time (PT) and the activated partial thromboplastin time (APTT) are the tests generally used that examine special proteins to evaluate most of the clotting factors, which measure their ability to help blood clot. Factors involved in the intrinsic pathway of coagulation are evaluated by the TTP while the PT evaluates the extrinsic pathway, both of which overlap in common pathway factors.

When bleeding begins, the body initiates a series of activities that help the blood to clot, which is called the coagulation cascade. This test is performed to determine the tendency of the blood to clot by measuring if there is a blood clotting disorder and also to know the status of any treatment, in this case if you are taking an anticoagulant such as warfarin or if you have liver failure.

For this test the sample with the light blue cap is required, the tube contains sodium citrate, causing the blood to be anticoagulated. The citrate functions as a calcium chelator.

10.8.1 Prothrombin time

The PT prothrombin time is the time it takes for a patient's plasma to clot when a reagent containing thromboplastin and phospholipids is added to it. This reagent binds to plasma factor VII and activates the so-called extrinsic coagulation pathway, which comprises factors VII, X, V and II. Factor II is prothrombin which, once activated, becomes thrombin which acts on fibrinogen to form fibrin. Any decrease in factors increases PT.

The exercise by which the prothrombin time is determined is by means of the coagulimetric method that measures the time it takes to form the clot, it works through the addition of the reagent to the patient's plasma, all this in the presence of calcium ions that initiates the activation of the extrinsic pathway of coagulation.

The international normalized ratio (INR) used in the treatment with oral anticoagulants may also often be requested, and became necessary due to the different sensitivity of the commercial thromboplastins used as reagent.

To standardize the results internationally, a committee of the World Health Organization (WHO) developed and recommended the use of the INR or International Normalized Ratio together with the prothrombin time (PT) in patients under anticoagulant therapy.

The International Sensitivity Index (ISI) is involved in the calculation of the INR because each commercial thromboplastin has an ISI that is obtained by comparing it with a WHO standard thromboplastin. The INR is a calculation that minimizes changes due to the reagents used and allows comparison of results between laboratories. Many laboratories now provide PT and INR results whenever a PT test is performed.

The reference values for Prothrombin Time is expressed in seconds ranging from 10-13.5 seconds and the Prothrombin Time ratio ranges from 0.8-1.2 seconds and for people on warfarin treatment, 2.0 to 3.0 seconds, although the INR may be higher in particular situations.

When any of the blood clotting factors are missing or not working properly, the PT varies and this is where it can be seen:

1. Increased by anticoagulants.

2. Enlarged in the deficit of coagulation factors II, V, VII and X, which are vitamin K-dependent or hepatic synthesis factors.

3. Lengthened due to various reasons such as hepatopathies (hepatitis), intestinal malabsorption or vitamin K deficiency.

4. Shortened in estrogen treatment, or by some prothrombin mutation.

5. A high or too low result in warfarin treatment due to wrong dosage of the drug.

An INR above 1.1 seconds indicates that anticoagulants are not being taken, i.e. the blood is clotting more slowly and may be due to bleeding disorders, disseminated intravascular coagulation, liver disease, low vitamin K levels, etc.

Having an INR between 2.0 and 3.0 seconds is ideal if you are on treatment with Waefarin, in order to prevent blood clots. An INR = 5 indicates that there is a high chance of bleeding, while an INR = 0.5 indicates that there is a high chance of having a clot.

10.8.2 Partial Thromboplastin Time

TTP measures the time it takes for a patient's plasma sample to clot when in contact with a reagent containing partial thromboplastin (phospholipids) in the presence of an activator and calcium, thus promoting the formation of thrombin from the plasma under study. The activator provides a surface that participates in a conformational change of plasma factor XII, resulting in its activation.

TTP is used for the study of factors of the intrinsic coagulation pathway in which factors XII, XI, IX, VIII, X, V and I (fibrinogen) are involved, giving prolonged values when one or more of them are not at normal levels, also for the monitoring of treatment with heparin or presence of lipid anticoagulant or other inhibitors.

The method by which TTP residuals are determined is coagulimetric. Where the patient's plasma is incubated with an optimal amount of phospholipids, here a negatively charged contact surface with a buffer initiates the activation of the intrinsic coagulation pathway. After incubation at 37°C for a certain period of time, Cl2Ca is added to trigger the clotting process and the time required for clot formation is measured.

TTP values are expressed in seconds ranging from 20-33.5 in the laboratory.

The TTP is prolonged by deficiencies of factors such as factor XI, IX, VIII, X, V, prothrombin and fibrinogen, also in treatment with specific anticoagulants such as lupic, treatment with unfractionated heparin, etc.

An abnormal TPT result that is too long may be due to a disorder where the proteins that control clotting become overactive (disseminated intravascular coagulation), liver disease, difficulty absorbing nutrients from food (malabsorption), vitamin K deficiency and also when the individual is producing a type of autoantibody known as antiphospholipid antibodies; which interfere with the test. The interference occurs because these autoantibodies are directed against substances known as phospholipids, also used in the TTP reaction. Although antiphospholipid antibodies prolong the TTP, their presence in the body is associated with excessive clotting and therefore people who develop them are at increased risk of clot formation. TTP can be useful in the evaluation of individuals with signs and symptoms of excessive clotting or antiphospholipid syndrome.

10.8.3 Equipment used

The equipment used in the laboratory is a semi-automatic coagulation analyzer for PT and TTP using the optical-mechanical principle for the detection of a clot. Through the use of the magnetic method to detect when clot formation occurs, measuring by the principle of nephelometry that detects clot formation.

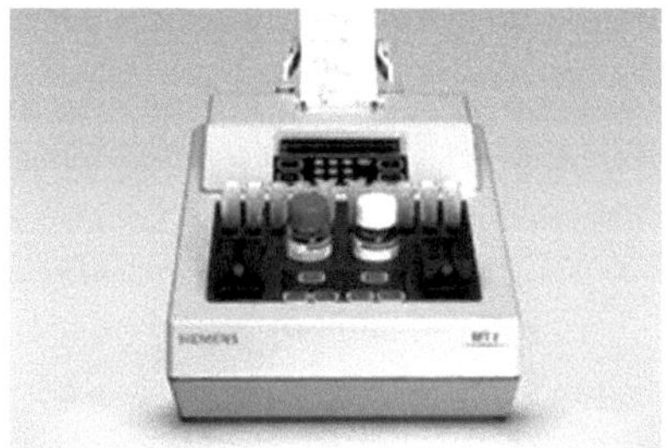

Figure 20. Semiautomated equipment for coagulation tests.

Mechanical detection is based on the increase in plasma viscosity when fibrin formation occurs using a cuvette with an incorporated steel ball. The principle consists of measuring the amplitude variations of the oscillation of a ball in the cuvette by means of electromagnetic sensors during the coagulation process.

The ball is held in position in the cuvette by the action of a magnetic magnet. With the addition of the reagent, the cuvette starts to rotate around its longitudinal axis and the ball is held in place by the magnetic field. The formation of fibrin displaces the ball from its original position and this change of position is registered by a sensor that automatically registers the time of clot formation. These devices also make an optical detection of the clot.

Optical detection is based on a beam of light located under the cuvette passing directly through the sample to the detector. When the fibrin mesh is formed the light beam is deflected and can be detected at a certain angle from the original beam position. This is where the stopwatch stops when the amount of transmitted or scattered light reaches a predetermined level. The difference between the transmitted or scattered light before and after clot formation is usually proportional to the amount of fibrin. A calculation algorithm uses these variations to deduce and accurately determine the coagulation times in the cuvette (17).

To determine the TP and TTP it is necessary to add several reagents to the cuvette required by the equipment.

For the determination of these tests it is required to use the equipment and perform the following procedure:

- To perform PT, first select the test to be performed on the device.

- Place the pellet plus 50 µL of plasma in the cuvette.

- Start the incubation process for a period of 60 seconds.

- Add 100 µL of TP reagent prewarmed to 37°C.

- Wait for the result issued by the equipment

- To perform TTP, first select the test to be performed on the device.

- Place in the cuvette the pellet plus 50 µL of plasma.

- Add 50 µL of TTP reagent prewarmed to 37°C.

- Start the incubation process for a period of 180 seconds.

- Place 50 µL of preheated 37°C calcium chloride in the cuvette.

- Wait for the result issued by the equipment.

11. Blood chemistry

In the area of blood chemistry we work with the blood serum, separating by centrifugation the cellular package of the serum, and it is here where all the components are dissolved to perform blood chemistry. Blood chemistry is the study by which through the metabolism of the body is analyzed the functioning of certain organs such as the liver and kidneys, thus allowing the physician to provide information about the conditions of the body's metabolism.

The El Carmen clinical analysis laboratory receives requests for blood chemistry comprising 3 and 6 elements. Below is a description of each of the tests performed in the laboratory.

11.1 Glucose

Glucose is the main source of energy in living beings. For this reason it is a fundamental metabolite in biological processes, it is a sugar that provides necessary energy to tissues and cellular metabolism. It is obtained through food, where it is stored mainly in the liver, which plays a major role in maintaining blood glucose levels (glycemia).

When sugar is ingested and rises in the blood, the hormone insulin is immediately released from the pancreas, specifically from the pancreatic β-cells (islets of langergans), allowing glucose to enter the cells so that glucose levels remain normal.

The main reason why diabetes mellitus originates is when insulin is insufficient, which is why glucose accumulates in the blood generating a constant situation, causing a series of complications at the cellular level, directly affecting all organs. Hyperglycemia and diabetes may not cause symptoms in the early stages. A fasting blood glucose test is almost always done to detect diabetes. The most common test performed in the laboratory is the determination of basal glycemia, which allows to determine the values of glucose in the blood, and for this it is convenient to perform it first thing in the morning, after 8 hours of fasting.

Diabetes Mellitus is a chronic degenerative, incurable but controllable disease that affects 15% of the world's population. Of this proportion of the population, Diabetes Mellitus Type 1 accounts for 10%, while Diabetes Mellitus Type 2 accounts for 85% (18) (19).

The way to diagnose Diabetes Mellitus is through the signs and symptoms it generates, such as:

- Hyperglycemia

- Arterial hypertension

- Polydipsia (need to drink)

- Polyuria (excess urine)

- Polyphagia (increased need to eat)

- Fatigue

- Weight loss

- Blurred vision

- Infections

- Poor healing

However, on many occasions, type 2 Diabetes Mellitus is asymptomatic, so in order to confirm or rule out the presence of this disease, stimulus response type tests have been developed. The best known of these tests is the Oral Glucose Tolerance Curve (OGTT).

Glucose analysis measures the amount in concentration of glucose present in the blood in order to study the possible presence of diabetes mellitus. As it is a very complex disease with great health repercussions, it is a very discriminating and useful test that is routinely used. Quantitative determination has been the subject of many studies and the literature offers various analysis techniques that vary according to different factors such as the nature of the sample, glucose contents and experimental feasibility.

According to the American Diabetes Association (ADA), fasting glucose test results are sufficient to diagnose diabetes mellitus. On the other hand, the World Health Association WHO recommends basing the diagnosis on the glycemia obtained 2 hours after an oral load of 75 g of glucose.

Diabetes Mellitus can be diagnosed by three different methods, and each of them must be confirmed within three days by any of the three methods:

- Basal glycemia in venous plasma equal to or greater than 126 mg/dl without caloric intake at least 8 hours prior to sampling.

- Random glycemia in venous plasma equal to or greater than 200 mg/dl in the presence of diabetic syndrome (polyuria, polyphagia, polydipsia, unexplained weight loss) random glycemia is glycemia at any time of the day, regardless of the time of the last meal.

- Venous plasma glycemia equal to or greater than 200 mg/dl at 2 hours after oral overload of 75 grams of glucose.

One of the methods currently used at the clinical and research level is the determination of basal glycemia, which is important to evaluate glucose levels in the first hour of the morning, after 8 hours of fasting, by taking a venous blood sample through the determination that is performed in the plasma by enzymatic methods.

The most common causes for which this test is requested are:

- Age over 45 years old

- Elevated blood sugar level in a previous test

- High blood pressure

- High cholesterol levels

- Women diagnosed with gestational diabetes

- Not being physically active

- Overweight or obesity

- General check-up routine

A high fasting result near the 70-110 mg/dl range means impaired glucose, a type of prediabetes. A level that exceeds the limits means that you have impaired fasting glucose, a type of prediabetes. A higher result almost always means diabetes is present. And if you do a random blood glucose test: A level at or above 200 mg/dl means you have diabetes.

A high result may be due to:

- Hyperthyroidism

- Pancreatic cancer

- Swelling and inflammation of the pancreas (pancreatitis)

A lower than normal blood glucose level (hypoglycemia) may be due to:

- Hypopituitarism (a disorder of the pituitary gland)

- Hypothyroidism or adrenal gland

- Tumor of the pancreas (insulinoma - very rare)

- Very little food

- Too much insulin or other diabetes medications

- Liver or kidney disease

- Weight loss after weight loss surgery

- Vigorous exercise

11.2 Urea

Urea is the body's final waste product of protein metabolism resulting from protein degradation. It is synthesized and carried out by the liver, passing into the bloodstream and being filtered by the kidneys to be excreted and carried to the bladder where urea is eliminated through urine.

Its formation is understood by means of a complex process in the organism. It begins through food; when food is ingested, once inside the organism it begins to degrade by means of enzymatic methods through digestion, where proteins are separated into amino acids, generating processes where proteins suffer the loss of nitrogen, which is released in the form of ammonium ion, it is there where the ammonium finally joins other molecules to produce urea, which must later be filtered in the kidney, as long as it is working properly.

The measurement of the urea level in the blood allows to identify a dysfunction of the kidneys, particularly a renal insufficiency. When there is an increase in the urea concentration in the bloodstream, it indicates that the kidneys are not performing their functions properly, probably because there is a renal lesion that disturbs the excretory function (20).

Normal reference values range from 10 to 50 mg/dl, these vary depending on some factors:

- When dehydration occurs, there is extra-renal azoemia (presence of nitrogen in the blood) (blood purification process), with high levels that are easily relieved by hydrating the body.

- When blood urea levels exceed 100 mg/dL of urea nitrogen, mental depression, drowsiness and electrolyte imbalance set in, and if the increase persists, uremic coma, usually irreversible, is reached.

- In normal pregnancy, blood urea levels are generally low.

- The urea level may be elevated during prolonged exertion or following high-protein diets. Also in case of heart failure, dehydration and during a postoperative phase. In elderly people, urea levels are usually relatively high.

As a precautionary measure it is important to mention that normal urea values differ according to the technique used by the laboratories, the results cannot constitute a diagnosis. It is therefore necessary to consult a physician for a correct interpretation and to prescribe the most appropriate treatment. All this means that the kidneys are not performing their functions properly.

Normal urea values in an adult person are between 10 and 50 mg/dl, values higher than 100 mg/dl are due to renal failure that should be treated immediately because high urea in the blood is dangerous to health and even fatal.

Increase in blood urea:

- Dehydration.

- Kidney problems, such as kidney stones due to renal failure.

- Very high protein diet.

Uremia can cause high blood urea, because metabolic wastes accumulate and the kidney becomes unable to process it all. Uremia is a set of respiratory, digestive, cerebral and circulatory symptoms caused by the accumulation of toxic products in the blood, when these cannot be eliminated by the kidney.

11.3 Creatinine

The metabolism of creatinine formation takes place in the following way, it starts with the amino acids glycine arginine and methionine that synthesize creatine in the liver, this molecule is necessary to obtain energy, all this in order to carry out the muscular metabolism. Creatine travels throughout the bloodstream and is distributed in all muscle cells, there we can find it in 98% of the totality of the whole organism. When it reaches the muscle and a muscle contraction occurs, creatine fulfills the function of being a molecule that participates in the formation of energy, performing a phosphorylation process where it is converted into phosphocreatine, and causing the loss of phosphorus, thus culminating the creatinine molecule, this is the final product of metabolism for the formation of creatinine. Only 2% percent of this substance is converted daily into creatinine, generating a waste product of the organism, in this process creatinine travels from the muscles through the bloodstream to the kidney, and here it is filtered and excreted mainly by the kidney through the urine, and only a small part through the feces. (21)

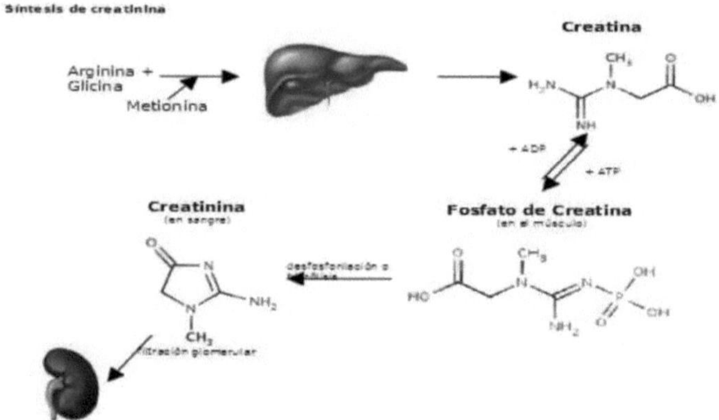

Figure 21. Synthesis of creatinine.

Creatinine is a constant waste substance and there is a direct relationship that depends on the muscular mass, for its elimination it is filtered through the kidney by the glomeruli, and eliminated through the urine. Once creatinine passes into the blood it is not reused and is constantly excreted, whereas creatine is reabsorbed by the tubules, which explains why only traces of this metabolite appear in the urine.

The determination of serum creatinine is a very specific and sensitive essential diagnostic test, since it indicates quite reliably information on the failures that allow detecting the state of renal function, i.e. if the kidneys do not work properly, they do not eliminate creatinine correctly, and therefore it accumulates in the blood. That is why creatinine is included in the blood tests that are commonly performed, warning of a possible dysfunction and even before the symptoms appear.

The normal range is between 0.6 and 1.1 md/dL for women and 0.7 and 1.3 mg/dL for men. The greater the renal function impairment, the higher the serum creatinine value. A normal concentration is proportional to the factor in relation to muscle mass. Adults with much greater muscle mass may have higher blood creatine, while the elderly population may have less creatine than normal. A very high concentration of creatinine in the blood indicates the need to undergo dialysis in order to remove all waste substances from the blood.

•   Elevated levels: renal failure, chronic nephritis, urinary tract obstruction, muscle mass (gigantism, acromegaly, myasthenia gravis, muscular dystrophy, poliomyelitis), congestive heart failure, shock, dehydration, rhabdomyolysis.

•   Decreased levels: people with short stature, decreased muscle mass, advanced or severe liver disease, inadequate protein diet, pregnancy (18).

11.4 Uric acid

Uric acid is a nitrogenous compound resulting from the catabolism of purine (a basic component of deoxyribonucleic acid DNA). The purine nucleotides are first degraded to hypoxanthine and xanthine as intermediate products, and finally oxidized to uric acid by the action of the enzyme xanthinoxidase. The formation of uric acid takes place mainly in the liver, which, like the intestinal mucosa, has a high xanthinoxidase activity.

Most of the uric acid dissolves in the blood and travels to the kidneys. Here uric acid is excreted in large amounts through the kidney and from there it is excreted through the urine (75%) and to a lesser extent through the intestine and feces (25%).

If the body produces too much uric acid or it is not eliminated in sufficient quantities and uric acid levels are high, it triggers hyperuricemia causing gout or kidney disease. Hyperuricemia is a disorder that occurs as a consequence of inadequate hepatic metabolism of nucleoproteins, the end product of which is uric acid. These disorders translate, at the organic level, into an increase of uric acid in the blood, which, in turn, can form crystalline deposits in the subcutaneous cellular tissue and joint capsules. The causes of hyperuricemia can be hyperproduction (patients with a catabolic enzyme deficit) or decreased uric acid excretion (e.g. renal insufficiency).

Many patients with hyperuricemia remain asymptomatic throughout their lives, but this likelihood decreases as the degree and duration of hyperuricemia increases. These patients should be treated if uricemia and uricosuria are elevated. The asymptomatic phase of hyperuricemia ends with the first attack of gouty arthritis or renal uric acid stones. The acute arthritic attack is triggered by the precipitation of uric acid in the form of urate crystals around the joints, in the cartilage, tendons, ligaments and in the cooler peripheral areas (fingers, ears). The most frequent localization is the first joint of the foot. In addition to localized inflammation, fever and other systemic effects derived from the inflammatory process may also occur.

Gout is characterized by an increase in the concentration of uric acid in the blood that the body is not able to eliminate through urine (by filtration in the kidneys), and this causes it to accumulate in the form of crystals of insoluble salts which are the urates, in certain joints interacting with the complement, coagulation, quinines and plasminogen systems, starting the respective enzymatic cascade that generates numerous molecules with inflammatory effect. This affection of the joints can eventually lead to chronic arthritis. In addition, the increased concentration of uric acid in the blood can cause kidney stones in the kidney because the pH of urine is acidic, and uric acid tends to be in acidic form, and very poorly soluble, tends to form crystals that can precipitate in the renal tubules causing renal insufficiency. A decrease in renal excretion of uric acid may be due to an idiopathic defect (22).

The risk of suffering and having an increase in the elevation of the level of uric acid or gout is mainly the hereditary factor without having committed excesses in terms of drinking or eating. Therefore, people who have a family member with hyperuricemia or gout present a higher risk of suffering from the disease. For this reason, it is recommended that individuals with a family history undergo an analytical control to know their blood uric acid values.

In general, hyperuricemia is a chronic disease that can be alleviated or controlled by maintaining an adequate diet. In not very severe hyperuricemia, diet together with good hydration may be sufficient to reach normal uric acid values, but in other cases, when purine metabolism is very affected, not only diet is necessary, but it must also be accompanied by pharmacological treatment.

The parameters for normal uric acid concentrations are in the blood reference range of 1.5 to 6.0 mg/dl in women and 2.5 to 7.0 mg/dl in men.

Factors that exceed the above mentioned limits may be due to: gout, congenital genetic enzymeopathy of purine metabolism, alcoholism, leukemia, metastatic cancer, multiple myeloma, hyperlipoproteinemia (diet rich in purines due to meat intake), anticancer chemotherapy, diabetes mellitus, renal insufficiency, dehydration, diuretic therapy, acidosis, advanced age, etc.

Lower levels may be due to: low purine diet, Wilson's disease, Fanconi's syndrome, lead poisoning, yellow liver atrophy.

11.5 Cholesterol

Cholesterol is the precursor of an indispensable element in the production of steroids, synthesis of female hormones (estrogens), main component of bile excretion, vitamin D, active catalyst of cellular exchanges, actively intervening in the synthesis of androgens and indispensable in the formation of cellular membranes. Chemically constituted by carbon, hydrogen, oxygen, phosphorus, among other elements.

The diet can provide a variable amount of cholesterol of exogenous origin, coming from the diet that is absorbed in the gastrointestinal tract and reaches the hepatocyte in the chylomicron remnants. Endogenous cholesterol, on the other hand, is synthesized in the liver in the hepatic cell from acetyl-CoA from sugar, fatty acids and amino acids, where almost all body cells are also capable of producing a quantity of endogenous cholesterol. In general, the body can manufacture all the cholesterol it needs, but in most individuals between 20% and 40% of cholesterol comes from food. Both endogenous and dietary cholesterol are involved in several important processes. (23)

There are two types of lipoproteins in the body: high-density lipoproteins and low-density lipoproteins. Cholesterol is carried in the blood by molecules called lipoproteins, in the form of macromolecular aggregates. The three main types of lipoproteins are classified according to their density:

•	Low-density lipoproteins (LDL) or "bad cholesterol" cause arterial disease. LDL transports cholesterol from the liver to cells throughout the body and can cause harmful accumulation in the coronary arteries leading to arteriosclerosis. Its plasma value should be less than 100 mg/dL.

•	High-density lipoproteins (HDL) or "good cholesterol", which are larger in size and higher in density, prevent arterial disease. HDL carries cholesterol away from the cells and returns it to the liver where it is broken down and eliminated as body waste, thus reducing arterial and coronary risks. Normal levels should not be higher than 40 mg/dL.

•	VLDL (low density lipoprotein) is a fat that shapes the organism as an organic reserve and forms part of what we know as triglycerides. Its normal levels fluctuate between 5 and 40 mg/dL.

The plasma cholesterol concentration in healthy individuals is 100 to 200 mg/dL. Increased plasma cholesterol levels are a cause of morbidity and mortality from cardiovascular disease and represent a serious health hazard. The deposition of cholesterol in the arterial wall is responsible for the formation of atheroma plaques causing the interruption of the correct blood flow, which can cause the organs to stop receiving oxygen and nourishment, which is why it is therefore evident the need for careful regulation to ensure that all metabolic destinations of cholesterol do not generate any pathology, which can cause even a heart attack or stroke (stroke).

The cholesterol level increases with age and in people over 70 years old, the normal figure is between 150-210. Above 200 mg/dL it should be controlled. At 220 mg/dL the coronary risk, which depends on genetic factors, diet, lifestyle, HDL concentration, etc. (18).

Increased levels may be associated with: hypothyroidism, uncontrolled diabetes, obesity, excessive caloric intake, nephrotic syndrome, cholesterol-rich diet, hypertension, atherosclerosis, stress, nephrosis, etc.

Decreased levels can result in: malnutrition, hyperthyroidism, pernicious anemia, liver disease.

If the diet we consume is high in "bad cholesterol", it begins to accumulate in the arteries that carry the blood, where it is stored and formed, which will eventually lead to atherosclerosis.

Most of the risk factors can be prevented, it is only necessary to modify eating habits and avoid the consumption of red meat, fried foods, large amounts of oil, and start with the consumption of almonds, nuts, avocado, fish and increase daily physical activity.

11.6 Triglycerides

Triglycerides are esters of glycerin or glycerol that constitute energy reserves in mammals. They are fatty compounds whose main function is to transport energy to the depot organs.

In general, fats are made up of mixed acylglycerols, i.e. the fatty acids that esterify glycerin are usually different, and when the proportion of saturated fats predominates, they are solid, and when there are more unsaturated fats, they are liquid.

The fats that we ingest in the diet are absorbed by the intestinal velocities and are used in small proportion for the direct supply of energy and are usually stored in the adipose tissue, reaching about 20% of weight in men and 25% in women, increasing its content with age, in general. And this reserve fat in the body does not necessarily come from fat consumption, but also from glucose from sugars and starches and also from amino acids if protein is taken in excess. When the liver and muscle glycogen stores are full, carbohydrates are stored in the form of triglycerides, and can be produced in the liver or come from the diet.

Normal blood triglyceride values range from 30-165 mg/dl, a higher value outside the range established by the laboratory is called hypertriglyceridemia. And it could generate the risk of developing cardiovascular problems. The risk of high triglyceride levels can trigger the development of atherosclerosis, which increases the likelihood of heart attack and stroke.

Lowering triglyceride levels is achieved by establishing a low-carbohydrate diet, avoiding refined sugars and sugary drinks. A high result of hypertriglyceridemia may be due to diabetes, obesity, tobacco smoking, alcohol intake and sedentary lifestyle (23).

11.7 Spectrophotometry

The equipment used in blood chemistry tests works on the principle of spectrophotometry, through the use of an equipment called spectrophotometer where different reagents are required depending on the analyte to be measured. Colorimetric reactions originate in the equipment that allow and effectively facilitate the automated handling of the equipment.

Spectrophotometry is a technique used to determine the concentration of a substance in relation between the absorption of light by a compound and its concentration. In this technique, monochromatic light at a single wavelength is incident on a homogeneous medium, where part of the incident light is absorbed by the medium and part is transmitted, and the amount of radiant energy absorbed by the molecules of a sample is quantified as a function of specific wavelengths.

To make it clearer, we start by mentioning that there is a lamp that provides a light source that emits a beam directly into the diffraction grating, the diffraction grating works like a prism, this is where the equipment separates the light into different wavelengths, as the light reaches the grating it is rotated so that only a specific desired wavelength reaches the exit slit, this is then where the light interacts in the compartment containing the sample to be analyzed. At this point a detector measures the transmittance and absorbance of the sample where transmittance refers to the amount of light that passes completely through the sample and hits the detector, and absorbance is a measurement of the light that is absorbed by the sample. Finally, the detector has the function of electronically measuring the intensity of the light that is transmitted through the sample in order to convert all the information and display it on a digital screen.

The blood chemistry equipment is used on a daily basis, so the following aspects must be taken into account:

1.   Switch on the equipment and check that the system is working properly.

2.   Remove the reagent carousel from the refrigerator to allow the reagents to cool down.

3.   Check that the carousel has sufficient quantity of reagents, if it is the case to replace the missing reagent quantity.

4.   Calibrate the equipment based on the use of controls.

5. Fill the cups with the serum to be analyzed in the wells corresponding to the previous labeling.

6. Select in the equipment the different tests to be evaluated in each serum sample.

7. Once all of the above points have been completed, the samples are processed.

8. Filling in the mandatory fields for each patient such as date, age, sex, name, physician requesting the exam, folio number, etc.

9. Obtaining the results.

10. Printing of results for each patient on letterhead.

11. Perform maintenance before shutting down the equipment.

11.8 Chemical reactions of blood chemistry

The glucose present in the sample is catalyzed by glucose oxidase (GOD), which is oxidized to gluconic acid and formation of hydrogen peroxide (H_2O_2). The hydrogen peroxide produced, phenol and 4-aminoantipyrine (4-AA) in the presence of peroxidase (POD) are condensed by the action of hydrogen peroxide, forming a red quinonaimine proportional to the concentration of glucose in the sample.

$$\text{Glucose} + H_2O + O_2 \xrightarrow{\text{GOD}} \text{Gluconic} + H_2O_2$$

$$H_2O_2 + 4\text{-AA} + \text{Phenol} \xrightarrow{\text{POD}} \text{red quinonaimine} + H_2O$$

The urea present in the sample is specifically hydrolyzed by urease decomposing it and producing carbon dioxide and ammonia; this reacts with phenol and hypochlorite in an alkaline medium producing indophenol with a blue color that is determined colorimetrically.

$$\text{Urea} + H_2O_2 \xrightarrow{\text{urease}} 2\,NH_3 + CO_2$$

$$NH_3 + \text{phenol} + NaCl \longrightarrow \text{infophenol} + NAD+ + H_2O$$

The creatinine present in the sample reacts with the picrate in an alkaline medium, reacting with the picrate ions to form a reddish colored complex where the intensity of the color formed is proportional to the concentration of creatinine in the sample tested.

The rate of formation of the complex is measured in short initial periods, thus avoiding interference from other compounds, and is quantified by photometric reading.

pH > 12

Creatinine +Picric acid ---------------- → red picrate-creatinine complex

37°C

Uric acid is oxidized by the action of the specific enzyme uricase to allantoin and hydrogen peroxide which in the presence of enzyme peroxidase (POD), 4-aminophenazone (4-AF) and 2-4 Dichlorophenol Sulfonate (DCPS) forms a pinkish compound proportional to the concentration of uric acid in the sample.

Uricase

Uric acid + 2 H_2O + O_2 -------------------→ Allantoin + CO_2 + 2 H_2O_2

POD

2 H_2O_2 + 4-AF + DCPS -----→ red quinonaimine + 4⅛O

The intensity of red quinonaimine formed is proportional to the concentration of uric acid present in the sample tested.

The method for the determination of total cholesterol in serum is based on the use of three enzymes: cholesterol esterase (CE), cholesterol oxidase (CO) and peroxidase (POD). In the presence of the latter, the mixture of phenol and 4-aminoantipyrine (4-AA) are condensed by the action of hydrogen peroxide, forming a colored quinonaimine proportional to the concentration of cholesterol in the sample.

CE

Esterified cholesterol + H_2O -------------→ Cholesterol + Fatty acids

CO

Cholesterol + ½ O_2+ H_2O ------→ Cholestenone + H_2O_2

H_2O_2

2 H_2O 4-AA + Phenol -----------------→ Quinonaimine + 4 H_2O

For triglyceride determinations, triglycerides are incubated with lipoprotein lipase (LPL) which releases glycerol and free fatty acids. Glycerol is phosphorylated by glycerol phosphate dehydrogenase (GPO) and ATP in the presence of glycerol kinase (GK) to produce glycerol-3-phosphate (G3P) and adenosine-5-diphosphate (ADP). G3P is then converted to dihydroxyacetone phosphate (DAP) and hydrogen peroxide (H_2O_2) by GPO. Finally, hydrogen peroxide (H_2O_2) reacts with 4-aminophenazone (4-AF) and p-chlorophenol, a reaction catalyzed by peroxidase (POD) giving a red coloration:

LPL

61

$$\text{Triglycerides} + H_2O \longrightarrow \text{Glycerol} + \text{Free fatty acids}$$

$$\text{Glycerol kinase (GK)}$$

$$\text{Glycerol} + ATP \longrightarrow G3P + ADP$$

$$\text{GOP}$$

$$G3P + O_2 \longrightarrow DAP + H_2O_2$$

$$\text{POD}$$

$$H_2O_2 + 4\text{-AF} + p\text{-Chlorophenol} \longrightarrow \text{Quinone} + H_2O$$

The intensity of the color formed is proportional to the concentration of triglycerides present in the sample tested.

12. Serology

Serology is the branch of immunology that studies the interactions of an antigen with an antibody. With the purpose of its application in clinical diagnosis. Serological tests are used for the identification of unknown agents present in clinical specimens, where blood serum is isolated and brought into contact with test reagents containing known concentrations of antigen or antibodies reacting antigen-antibody. And thus, allowing to evidence information about infections, immune response and biological components.

Results are not reported in concrete units but in relative units, expressed as positive or negative.

12.1 C-reactive protein (CRP)

C-reactive protein (CRP) has been considered and used as a systemic marker of inflammation that occurs as a consequence of the organism's response to any type of aggression, generally by an infectious agent; therefore, its determination has a certain diagnostic value. Traditionally, the magnitude of CRP concentration has been used for the diagnosis and monitoring of some autoimmune and infectious diseases; however, it has recently been identified as a predictor of cardiovascular risk.

Plasma protein C is secreted in the liver (on hepatocytes), inducing them to produce protein C. It increases when acute inflammation, infection or tissue degradation occurs in the body. Increasing plasma concentrations of proinflammatory cytokines such as interleukin IL-6 (produced by macrophages, endothelial cells and T lymphocytes) promote its synthesis and exert a proinflammatory action.

Pentraxins are a subfamily of acute phase reactants, characterized by having a multimeric cyclic structure, and some of its components are C-reactive protein, whose synthesis increases extraordinarily in inflammatory processes (24).

Their physiological values vary from laboratory to laboratory, but are usually less than 10mg/L. The physician can also perform a highly sensitive test, called the High Sensitivity CRP Test, to determine the patient's risk of possible heart disease.

Currently, serum levels greater than 10 mg/L are considered to be a marker indicating the presence of an acute infectious response. Levels below 1 mg/L are found in healthy individuals, and the presence of CRP in amounts between 1 and 10 mg/L are considered to be related to an increased risk of developing, in the indefinite term, coronary heart disease.

According to the American Heart Association:

• There is a low risk of developing cardiovascular disease if the CRP level is less than 1 mg/L.

• There is an average risk of suffering cardiovascular disease if CRP levels range between 1 and 3 mg/L.

• There is a high risk of cardiovascular disease if CRP levels are higher than 3 mg/L.

These values may be increased in cases of: Acute rheumatoid arthritis, rheumatic fever, certain autoimmune diseases such as lupus, Myocardial or pulmonary infarction, Bacterial infections, problems with rejection in transplants, infection, cancer, etc.

In the laboratory, the direct method is used by means of latex agglutination for qualitative and semi-quantitative tests, depending on the interpretation of the results.

For the qualitative test it is necessary to temper the reagents and resuspend them before use. We need first to place on the plate 20µl of test serum in the first circle, 20µl of positive control (+) in the second circle and 20µl of negative control (-) in the third circle. Add to each of the three circles 20µl of the anti-PCR reagent and mix homogeneously with wooden sticks taking care to always use only one stick for each circle. Once the procedure is finished, the plate is placed in the bortex and the stopwatch is triggered for 3 minutes, after this time and by means of a suitable light, the results are interpreted observing some type of agglutination where the problem sample was placed.

Negative reaction: homogeneous suspension without any visible change as in the negative control.

Positive reaction: weak or intense agglutination macroscopically visible.

If the sample is positive, the semi-quantitative technique is used by dilutions. In this test six circles are used, in each of the six circles 20µL of solution already prepared by the kit are poured. In the first circle add 20µL of sample and mix homogeneously with the tip of the micropipette performing repeated aspirations and expulsions, once this step is done proceed to transfer 20 µL of the resulting mixture on the diluent of the second circle. Continue with the series of double dilutions until the sixth circle, discarding the 20 µL coming from it. The final dilutions obtained from each of the circles will be: 1:2, 1:4, 1:8, 1:16, 1:32, 1:64. Finally, add 20 µL of anti-PCR reagent to each of the six circles and mix homogeneously with wooden sticks, taking care to use only one stick for each circle. Once the procedure is finished, place the plate in the bortex and trigger the stopwatch for 3 minutes to interpret the results. Observe immediately with the help of a suitable light looking for any sign of agglutination. The titer of the sample corresponds to the maximum dilution that shows reactivity. The next dilution should be negative.

To report the final result of the semi-quantitative PCR method, it is calculated by means of a formula that takes into account the last titer where an agglutination is presented by a positive result, multiplying it by 6. At first sight it would be: 6 x PCR titer = mg/L. Its formula is: PCR (mg/l) = titer x sensitivity of the reaction (6 mg/l) and an example would be: the sample presents a titer of 1:2. Its PCR concentration is 2 x 6 = 12 mg/L.

The reference value considered normal in the laboratory is 6 mg/L.

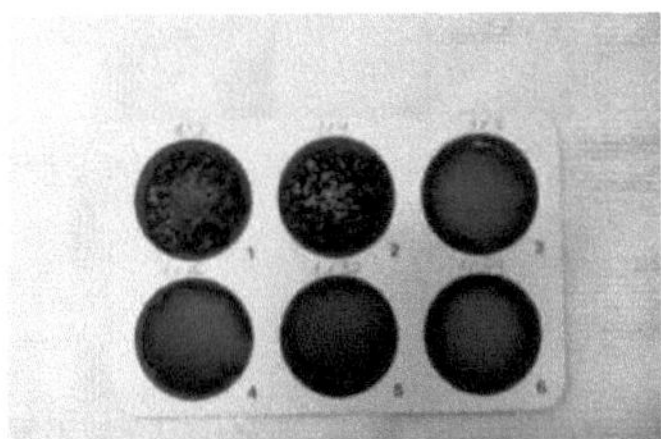

Figure 22. Agglutination of latex particles quantitative technique.

12.2 Rheumatoid factor

Rheumatoid factor refers to autoantibodies of different immunoglobulin classes directed primarily against specific sites of the fc region (constant fraction) of immunoglobulin molecules forming immunocomplexes capable of complement activation, which are constituted by IgM and IgG, where they are deposited in the synovial region and blood vessels of patients with rheumatoid arthritis. The alteration of the immune tolerance mechanisms triggers a persistent and exaggerated immune response manifested by the formation of autoreactive T-cell clones and the spontaneous production of autoantibodies directed against cellular structures or autoantigens.

Rheumatoid arthritis is a systemic, inflammatory and chronic disease localized in the joints. It is characterized by the activation of different synovial cell populations and the production of proinflammatory mediators such as cytosines, prostaglandins and proteases. It is generally considered to be an autoimmune disease.

Therapeutic measures can be taken to suppress the inflammatory manifestations of the disease and help reduce skeletal muscle dysfunction.

It is not yet clear and the antigens triggering the origin and pathogenesis of rheumatoid factor have not yet been identified. What is a fact is that the sera of patients diagnosed with rheumatoid arthritis present many autoantibodies, but only a few have pathogenic, diagnostic or prognostic value. Among them, the only one used in daily practice is rheumatoid factor, which is present in the serum of most patients with rheumatoid arthritis. Therefore, the tests used for the early detection of rheumatoid factor have an important clinical significance and will remain the main laboratory test for its diagnosis. Although there is a possibility of a seronegative result (25).

Patients with elevated concentrations have increased rheumatoid factor and immunoglobulin M, and are at risk of developing severe erosive joint disease with inflamed joints and extra-articular manifestations. Serum rheumatoid factor appears more commonly, with higher titers, in patients with chronic systemic disease; these antibodies are detected in approximately 70 to 80 percent of patients with rheumatoid arthritis.

The determination of rheumatoid factor in serum is carried out by the latex agglutination test method, where IgM antibody groups are detected by an immunological agglutination reaction. The Latex-FR Reagent is a suspension of polystyrene particles sensitized with human immunoglobulin, containing IgG immunoglobulins absorbed on the latex particles. By directly mixing the sample with the latex-FR reagent, the presence of rheumatoid factors (with anti-IgG capacity) causes agglutination of the latex particles, which is visualized macroscopically. These particles reveal the antigen-antibody relationship where the patient's rheumatoid factor forms a clear agglutination.

Rheumatoid factor results range from less than 0 - 40 UI/mL as a normal result, although there are lower titers that are low but suspicious, when the figures are higher than 20 40 80 160 or 320 UI/mL means that the greater the compatibility with the diagnosis of arthritis. False positives can also be found in patients with hyperlipidemic serum.

A low number which would be a normal result usually means that you do not have rheumatoid arthritis or Sjogren's syndrome. But also some people who actually have these conditions also have a low or relatively normal rheumatoid factor result.

Conversely, an abnormal result means that the test is positive, which means that higher levels of rheumatoid factor have been detected in your blood. The higher the level, the greater the likelihood that a condition is present.

People with the following diseases may also have higher levels of rheumatoid factor and for their diagnosis this test is not used, such as: infectious mononucleosis, hepatitis, tuberculosis, syphilis, leishmaniasis, healthy elderly adults etc.

In the laboratory, the direct method is used by means of latex agglutination for qualitative and semi-quantitative tests, depending on the interpretation of the results.

For the qualitative test it is necessary to temper the reagents and resuspend them before use. We first need to place 20µl of test serum in the first circle, 20µl of positive control (+) in the second circle and 20µl of negative control (-) in the third circle. Add to each of the three circles 20µl of FR-latex reagent and mix homogeneously with wooden sticks taking care to always use only one stick for each circle. Once the procedure is finished, the plate is placed in the bortex and the stopwatch is fired for 3 minutes, after this time and by means of a suitable light, the results are interpreted observing some type of agglutination where the problem sample was placed.

Negative reaction: uniform suspension with no visible change as in the negative control.

Positive reaction: weak or intense agglutination macroscopically visible.

If the sample is positive, the semi-quantitative technique is used by dilutions. In this test six circles are used, in each of the six circles 20µL of solution already prepared by the kit are poured. In the first circle add 20µL of sample and mix homogeneously with the tip of the micropipette performing repeated aspirations and expulsions, once this step is done proceed to transfer 20 µL of the resulting mixture on the diluent of the second circle. Continue with the series of double dilutions until the sixth circle, discarding the 20 µL coming from it. The final dilutions obtained from each of the circles will be: 1:2, 1:4, 1:8, 1:16, 1:32, 1:64. Finally, add 20 µL of FR-Latex reagent to each of the six circles and mix homogeneously with wooden sticks, taking care to use only one stick for each circle. Once the procedure is finished, place the plate in the bortex and trigger the stopwatch for 3 minutes to interpret the results. Observe immediately with the help of a suitable light looking for any sign of agglutination. The titer of the sample corresponds to the maximum dilution that shows reactivity. The next dilution should be negative.

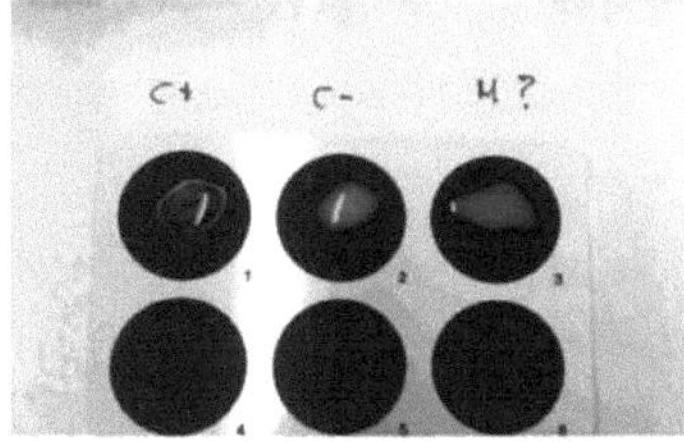

Figure 23. Rheumatoid factor qualitative technique.

12.3 Antistreptolysins

Antistreptolysins are antibodies directed against hemolysin "O" of beta-hemolytic streptococcus. The antistreptolysin test assesses antibodies to hemolysin "O". It is used to test for the presence of antibodies to streptolysin "O", one of a number of enzymes produced by streptococcus that have the power to destroy red blood cells.

Streptococci are a diverse group of catalase-negative, facultative aerobic, gram-positive cocci that cause various toxicological and pyogenic infections in humans. The most prominent of which is *Streptococcus pyogenes* which is the cause of the bacterium causing pharyngitis.

The antigenic composition of streptococci is complex, and has 18 group-specific carbohydrate antigens, nominated A through R, which are useful in classifying streptococci. Type A streptococci produce an enzyme called streptolysin "O" which has the ability to lyse hematopoiesis, behaving like an antigen. The organism reacts by producing neutralizing antibodies that appear between 8 to 30 days after the onset of the streptococcal infection.

Streptococci can generate an infection with certain strains of this species that leads to long-term rheumatic fever and glomerulonephritis. Immunopathology has not yet resolved the chronic nature of rheumatic fever, what is known is that group A streptococci contain M-proteins that generate protective antibodies that are antiphagocytic factors and increase the virulence of the streptococci. The M-protein cross-reacts with myosin of the heart and this leads to autoimmunity. Although the cell wall of group A streptococci is highly resistant to degradation in the host. These antigens persist for months causing diseases resembling arthritis and rheumatoid carditis.

Group A B C F and G streptococci produce many extracellular substances that can elicit protective immunity. Streptolysins O and S are cytoplasmic proteins that inhibit phagocytosis and killing by eukocytes. There are several proteinases including streptokinase and other degradative enzymes such as hyaluronidase and deoxyribonuclease, which increase the pathogenicity of the organism. During infection antibodies may be produced against all these factors.

The determination of anti-streptolysin antibodies is used systematically in many clinical laboratories in the diagnosis of infections such as group A β-hemolytic streptococcus (Streptococcus pyogenes), bacteria capable of invading the upper respiratory tract as well as other soft tissues. These microorganisms produce pharyngitis inducing the production of anti-streptolysin O antibodies, which can be detected in the laboratory by the agglutination method.

This is an easy to perform semi-quantitative serological agglutination test that determines the value of anti-streptolysin against streptolysin "O" antibodies. For the interpretation of the titers obtained in the determination of anti-streptolysin "O", the reference values of the commercial kit were used. The values in the laboratory are considered normal if their value is less than 200 IU/mL. This test will determine the individual's contact with streptococcus over a period of approximately six months.

Anti-streptolysin O antibodies are detected in serum by their reaction with streptolysin O (produced by β-hemolytic streptococci) adsorbed on inert latex support. Quantification of the antibodies is used for the diagnosis and treatment of diseases such as rheumatic fevers, acute glomerulonephritis, and other streptococcal infections. The anti-streptolysin "O" antibody is present in almost all people in low titers, because streptococcal infections are common. ASO-Latex is a slide agglutination technique for the qualitative and semi-quantitative detection of anti-streptolysin "O" in serum. Streptolysin "O" coated latex particles are agglutinated by antibodies present in the patient's sample. This causes the anti-streptolysin antibodies to react with the streptolysin producing a macroscopically visible agglutination.

For the qualitative test it is necessary to temper the reagents and resuspend them before use. We need first to place on the plate 20µl of test serum in the first circle, 20µl of positive control (+) in the second circle and 20µl of negative control (-) in the third circle. Add to each of the three circles 20µl of ASO-latex reagent and mix homogeneously with wooden sticks taking care to always use only one stick for each circle. Once the procedure is finished, the plate is placed in the bortex and the stopwatch is fired for 3 minutes, after this time and by means of a suitable light, the results are interpreted observing some type of agglutination where the problem sample was placed.

Negative reaction: uniform suspension with no visible change as in the negative control.

Positive reaction: weak or intense agglutination macroscopically visible.

If the sample is positive, the semi-quantitative technique is used by dilutions. In this test six circles are used, in each of the six circles 20µL of solution already prepared by the kit are poured. In the first circle add 20µL of sample and mix homogeneously with the tip of the micropipette performing repeated aspirations and expulsions, once this step is done proceed to transfer 20 µL of the resulting mixture on the diluent of the second circle. Continue with the series of double dilutions until the sixth circle, discarding the 20 µL coming from it. The final dilutions obtained from each of the circles will be: 1:2, 1:4, 1:8, 1:16, 1:32, 1:64. Finally, add 20 µL of ASO-Latex reagent to each of the six circles and mix homogeneously with wooden sticks, taking care to use only one stick for each circle. Once the procedure is finished, place the plate in the bortex and fire the stopwatch for 3 minutes to interpret the results. Observe immediately with the help of a suitable light looking for any sign of agglutination. The titer of the sample corresponds to the maximum dilution that shows reactivity. The next dilution should be negative.

To interpret the results obtained from the semi-quantitative method of anti-streptolysin "O", the results are calculated by means of a formula where the last titer where agglutination is present is taken into account by means of a positive result. The approximate level of antistreptolysin "O" in the sample is calculated by the following formula: ASO (UI/ml) = titer x sensitivity of the reaction (200 UI/ml) Example: the sample has a titer of 1:2. The ASO level is 2 x 200 = 400 IU/ml.

Normal reference values are less than 200 UI/mL.

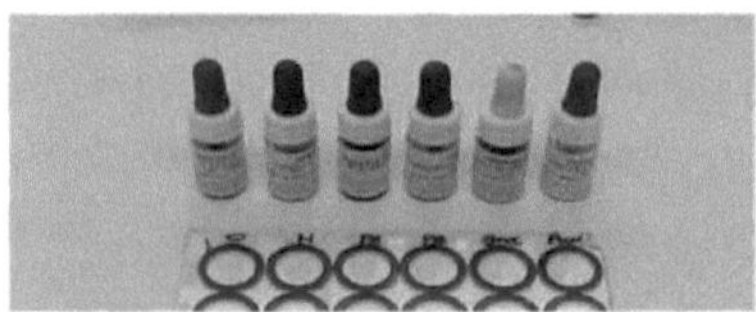

Figure 24. Material required to perform the antistreptolysin test.

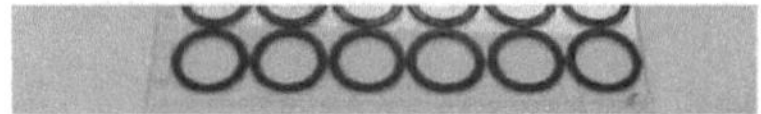

12.4 Febrile reactions

Febrile reactions are a set of tests that in developing countries such as Mexico, are used to diagnose diseases with temperature symptoms that cause fever due to infection by bacteria of various species, such as typhoid fever, brucellosis and rickettsiosis. In this test, febrile antigens are used to detect antibodies in the patient's serum against Salmonella, Brucella and Rickettsiae.

12.4.1 Salmonella

The transmission of Salmonella is through contaminated food and water causing typhoid fever, which is a highly prevalent infectious disease worldwide. *Salmonella* cause symptoms such as gastroenteritis, septicemia with lesions in various organs and the aforementioned typhoid fever.

It is detected in the laboratory by Widal's reaction in a serological method commonly used in the diagnosis of typhoid fevers, the reaction measures the serum titer against a suspension of known microorganism. Widal's reaction is a test based on the principle of antigen-antibody agglutination, where the presence of antibodies against the typhoid antigen H and O of *Salmonella typhi and* the paraphoid antigen A and B is determined.

12.4.2 Brucella

It is a zoonosis, that is, a disease transmitted from animals to humans caused by bacteria of the genus *Brucella*. This disease is acquired by ingesting contaminated food or maintaining close contact with livestock.

Brucellosis in humans is transmitted by ingestion of contaminated, unpasteurized milk, its products and derivatives, by contact with products, by-products and wastes such as tissues or excretions of sick animals, and by inoculation or inhalation of dust from corrals or slaughterhouses, where they are found. Brucellosis presents in most cases with anorexia, fever, weakness and chills, presenting undulatory febrile episodes, hence the name "undulant fever".

Its detection is through antibodies against *Brucella*, particularly due to *B. abortus, B. suis and B. melitenis*.

Its detection is by means of the Huddleson reaction, which is also a rapid agglutination reaction in a plate where decreasing amounts of the serum to be investigated are confronted with constant amounts of antigen and the presence or absence of agglutination is observed.

12.4.3 Rickettsiae

Rickettsiae are bacteria transmitted by vectors such as fleas, ticks and lice. In general, Rickettsiosis is considered a zoonosis, with the human being an accidental host. They are intracellular parasites, very sensitive and rarely survive outside the host, except for *Coxiella burnetii* (producer of Q fever) which is resistant to desiccation, heat and sunlight and is transmitted mainly by air. The rest is inoculated to the host directly through a bite in the dermis produced by the vector, by contamination of the bite with the feces of the insect or by inoculation of the mucous membranes with contaminated feces of the same. Causing symptoms such as fever, headache, skin eruptions, abdominal pain, hepatomegaly, respiratory symptoms, etc.

Rickettsiosis can be divided into 3 main groups:

1. Typhus group: Epidemic typhus, due to *Rickettsia prowazekii*, transmitted by lice (Poulex ivitans) and endemic classical typhus, due to *Rickettsia typha* by flea.

2. Spotted fever group: *Rickettsia rickettsii*, involving more than 30 species, transmitted

mainly by mites and fleas (Rocky Mountain spotted fever).

3. Scrub typhus: Orientia tsutsugamushi, also called scrub typhus, transmitted by mites, other Rickettsiosis such as Q fever caused by *Coxiella burnetti* and Ehrlichiosis (caused by *Ehrlichia sp*).

For the qualitative test it is necessary to temper the reagents and resuspend them in the bortex before use. We first need to mark the glass plate with each of the reagents to be used, using the legends as follows: circle one H, circle two O, circle three A, circle four B, circle five HDD, and circle six Prot. Finishing this exercise to each one of the circles 50µl of serum problem will be added, also 50µ (one drop) of each one of the reactive antigens will be added, mix the antigen and the serum homogeneously with wooden sticks taking care to always use only one stick for each circle, once the procedure is finished the plate is placed in the shaker and the stopwatch is fired for 5 minutes, rest the glass plate in a resting state for another 5 minutes more to later begin to interpret the results. Search by means of a suitable light to interpret the results observing some type of agglutination where the problem sample was placed. Always take into account the use of the negative control and the positive control.

Negative reaction: uniform suspension with no visible change as in the negative control.

Positive reaction: weak or intense agglutination macroscopically visible.

The results are interpreted as positive or negative, depending on whether agglutination is present or not.

12.5 VDRL

This test is used to find antibodies against the bacterium called *Treponema pallidum* that causes syphilis, which is an infectious systemic disease transmitted by sexual contact, direct contact with lesions, direct contact with blood and from mother to child during pregnancy. Early detection and treatment of the disease is essential to avoid serious complications.

Usually this test is always accompanied by a blood typing test, these two tests are used quite frequently, as it is a prenuptial requirement in Mexico in order to obtain a marriage license. It is requested if you suspect or have signs and symptoms of a sexually transmitted disease. Also, screening for syphilis is a routine part of prenatal care during pregnancy. During the incubation period of the disease and up to 15 days after the onset of the syphilitic chancre, as antibodies have not yet been produced by the patient.

Syphilis is clinically characterized by a primary lesion, which is characterized by a painless ulcerative papule that heals on its own three weeks after contact, the secondary lesion is a rash affecting the skin and mucous membranes, fever, late skin lesions, indisposition, muscle pain, poor appetite. In tertiary or late syphilis, lesions affect organs such as the heart and CNS disorders.

Fetal infections occur most frequently in the case of untreated maternal primary infection. Clinical manifestations may be present at birth, but are usually seen between 3 weeks and 6 months of age. Symptoms of early congenital syphilis include skin rash, mucous membrane lesions, anemia and painful osteochondritis of long bones and can lead to death. Late manifestations of congenital syphilis include blindness, deformation of bones and teeth, deafness and gum. Thirty percent of in utero infections result in fetal death before birth (26).

The VDRL test (Venereal Disease Research Laboratory) or also known as the Wassermann test is a serological technique with sufficient sensitivity and specificity to complement the diagnosis of syphilis and to analyze the response to specific treatment. The VDRL procedure is an antigen-antibody flocculation reaction on glass or glass slide that is standardized for use in serum. Cardiolipin antigen is used to detect nonspecific antireponemal antibodies produced by the individual upon syphilitic infection.

From the beginning of the infection, certain substances called "reagins" appear in the serum of the infected individual, which react with cardiolipin, lecithin and cholesterol antigens. These reagins together with clinical signs are therefore the quickest and most useful procedures available for the diagnosis of syphilis. If the specimen contains reagin, it will bind to the antigen producing a visible flocculation. From the onset of infection, certain substances called "reagins" appear in the serum of the infected individual, which react with cardiolipin, lecithin and cholesterol antigens. These reagins together with clinical signs are therefore the quickest and most useful procedures available for the diagnosis of syphilis. If the specimen contains reagin, it will bind to the antigen producing a visible flocculation. Here the patient's serum is mixed with a fresh suspension of antigen, this mixture is shaken in a rotating manner and after a few minutes flocculation can be observed and the results can be expressed both qualitatively and quantitatively.

A negative test is normal and means that no syphilis antibodies have been seen in the blood sample. The screening test is more likely to be positive in the secondary and latent stages of syphilis. This test may give a false negative result during the early and late stages of the disease.

A positive test result may indicate that you have syphilis. If the test is positive, the next step is to confirm the results with a more specific test for syphilis.

For the qualitative VDRL test it is only necessary to place 50μL of test serum on the circle of the plate, plus 25μL of the reagent containing the VDRL antigen, mix homogeneously with a wooden stick and place the plate on the shaker to program the timer for a period of 8 minutes. Once this time has elapsed, the results are interpreted. Do not forget to mount the positive and negative controls.

Non-reactive: Homogeneous suspension with uniform particles.

Reagent: Large or small lumps depending on the degree of positivity.

The result is reported as positive or negative, according to the reaction obtained after performing the methodology indicated in the insert.

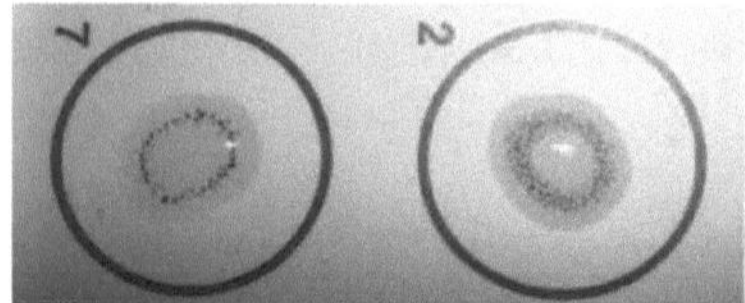

Figure 25. Positive result for VDRL.

12.6 Pregnancy test

This test is performed in order to detect the human chorionic gonadotropin hormone (HCG) from a blood or urine sample. This hormone is produced by the embryo and secreted by the placenta when conception occurs in the body. It is the hormone intended to indicate the presence or absence of an implanted embryo that can only be detected during pregnancy, and can even be identified as early as the sixth day after conception. The technique implemented in the laboratory is by means of the qualitative method.

All pregnancy tests are based on the detection of HCG, a hormone secreted by the placental trophoblast after fertilization of the ovum. HCG increases markedly, and serum levels are higher than urinary levels. After approximately one month of pregnancy, HCG concentrations are similar in both sample types.

The main function of the increase and production of HCG is to prevent the disintegration of the corpus luteum of the ovary, to produce more progesterone, which as its name says, is a fundamental hormone for pregnancy in human beings, it participates so that a good irrigation can be formed through vessels and capillaries and thus, sustain the growth of the fetus. Due to its high negative charge, hCG can repel the mother's immune cells, protecting the fetus during the first trimester.

HCG is composed of an alpha subunit and a beta subunit. The alpha subunit is the same in all glycoprotein hormones, while the beta subunit is specific to HCG. It is important to know that all pregnancy tests demonstrate the presence of HCG. (19)

The radioimmunoassay (RIA) technique used is simple, using only a strip that reads two lines to indicate the results. The test line uses a combination of elevated HCG levels. It is a reliable and highly sensitive blood test for the detection of the β-unit of HCG. Most tests use a monoclonal antibody specific to the β-subunit of HCG (βhCG). This method is so sensitive that pregnancy can be diagnosed even before the first missed period.

The assay is performed by dipping the test strip into a serum sample into the well and observing the formation of colored lines. The sample travels by the choromatographic method, by capillary action through the membrane to react with the color conjugate. Positive samples react with the color conjugate of the specific anti-hCG antibody to form a colored line in the test line region of the membrane. The absence of this color line suggests a negative result. To serve as a control for the procedure, a colored line will always appear in the region of the control line if the test has been performed correctly.

The identification of the hormone is based on a rapid lateral flow choromatographic immunoassay, using a conjugation of monoclonal-dye and polyclonal antibodies in solid phase to selectively identify hCG present in the samples. The sample from the absorbent portion migrates capillary across the strip. The antibody-dye conjugate binds to hCG forming an antibody-antigen complex. This complex binds to the anti-hCG antibody in the positive reaction zone producing a pink colored band.

In the absence of hCG, no band is observed in the positive reaction zone. The reaction mixture continues to migrate through the strip to the control zone. The free conjugate still binds to the reagents in the control zone forming a pink colored band, demonstrating the correct functioning of the test.

This test requires depositing 1 mL of serum sample in a small test tube, then inserting the HCG strip vertically into the sample for 10 minutes. Interpret the result as indicated on the insert.

A negative result: If only one colored transverse band appears in the upper white area (control band). And positive: In addition to the red transverse band (control) a second red or pink transverse band appears in the central white zone of the strip.

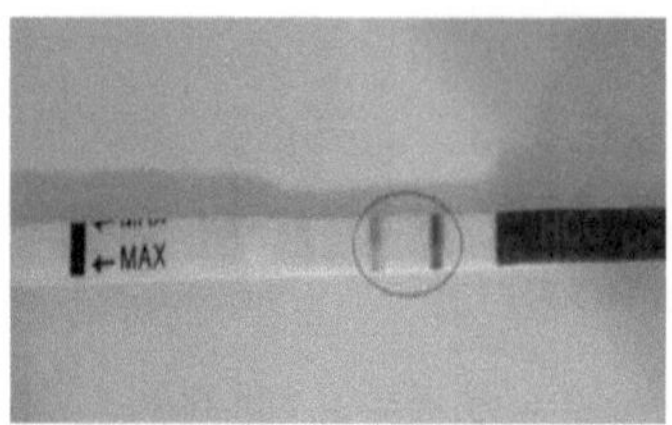

Figure 26. Positive test for HCG.

12.7 HIV1-2

The main mode of transmission of the acquired immunodeficiency virus is transmitted by the main sexual route worldwide. Two types of virus have been identified at the moment, but they are the same virus, with genetic differences that allow them to be classified into two different types. However, their genomes are only 45% similar; in fact, it is thought that HIV-2 originated in Africa from apes to man. The way both viruses act in the body is to attack our defenses, preventing our body from "defending" itself from external aggressions.

The HIV-1 virus is the most frequent and most infectious type, it is responsible for the worldwide AIDS epidemic and this type of virus evolves more slowly; therefore, its incubation period is longer, although both serotypes eventually cause Acquired Immune Deficiency Syndrome (AIDS).

The HIV-2 virus is associated with lower viral loads, it is less infectious and has a lower level of circulating virus, the disease it causes is less aggressive and its possibility of transmission is lower, which explains its reduced diffusion, in fact there are very few described cases of HIV-2. There is a lower probability of becoming infected with HIV-2, the transmission of HIV-2 through sexual contact is approximately 5 times lower than HIV-1.

HIV infection is associated at all stages with intense viral replication, mainly in lymphocytes and macrophages. Immunological mechanisms neutralize the new virions and regenerate the immune cells that are rapidly destroyed, achieving a balance between the amount of circulating virus, the viral load and the immune system, so that the virus carrier remains asymptomatic. After a variable period of time this equilibrium is broken, the viral concentration begins to increase and CD4 counts decline progressively. Immunological deterioration allows the appearance of various infections, both classical and opportunistic, and tumors, leading to AIDS and death in a variable period of time if not treated.

The basic aspect of the pathogenesis of HIV infection is the destruction of CD4+ helper lymphocytes with subsequent loss of immune system competence. It is an asymptomatic or symptomless infection for a variable period of up to about 8 years, due to the balance between viral replication and the patient's immune response. Subsequently, this balance is broken by increasing the viral load and deteriorating immune function, which allows the appearance of various infections, both classical and opportunistic, and tumors, leading to the stage of AIDS.

Antiviral treatment with associations of 3 antiretroviral drugs suppresses viral replication, making the viral load undetectable in more than 70% of cases, recovering qualitatively and quantitatively the immune response, decreasing progression and mortality due to AIDS.

Unfortunately, it is not possible to eradicate the viral genome from reservoir tissues, because during the initial stages of infection, reservoirs are established in the genome of latent cells that persist despite intense and long-lasting suppression of viral replication. Therefore, interruptions of antiviral treatment lead to the reappearance of circulating virus and new immunological and clinical deterioration.

The process in which the body decreases its natural defense until its complete disappearance and has nothing to fight any type of infectious disease is called acquired immunodeficiency syndrome AIDS, all due to the presence of the HIV virus in the body for a long time (27).

The diagnosis of HIV infection is made by the determination of specific antibodies against the virus, by ELISA technique.

The HIV-1 and HIV-2 Test Strip Assay is a comprehensive immunochromatographic test that employs a cocktail of antigens to detect the presence of anti-HIV 1 and 2 antibodies in serum, plasma or blood, where immobilized antigens are used to detect anti-HIV 1 and 2 antibodies with a high degree of sensitivity and specificity.

To perform this test, open an envelope to remove the cassette and place 1 drop of serum in the sample well plus 1 drop of buffer. Start the timer and wait 10 minutes to interpret the results. Observe the appearance of colored lines where the intensity of color in the test line zones (T1 and T2) will vary depending on the concentration of anti-HIV antibodies present in the sample, therefore any color tone in the detection line zone T1 and T2 should be considered positive.

In a positive result two different colored lines appear. There should always be one line in the control line zone (C) and one or two colored lines in the test line zones (T1 and/or T2).

A negative result is when a colored line appears in the control zone (C). No colored line appears in the test line zones (T1 and T2). An invalid result is when no control line appears.

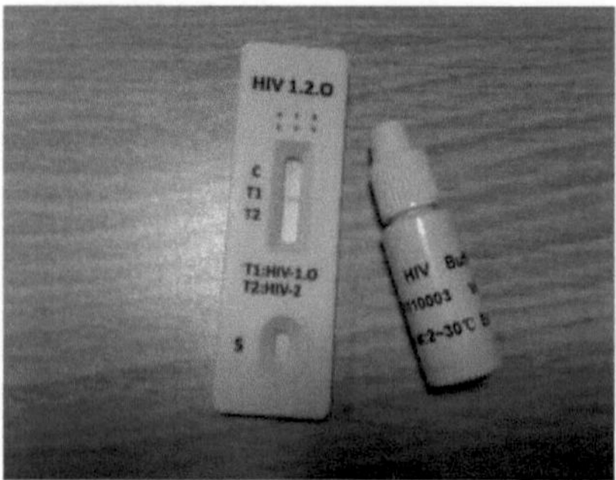

Figure 27. Positive test for HIV-1.

13. General Urine Test (GUR)

The general urine examination also called uroanalysis is the physical, chemical and microscopic evaluation of urine. The analysis consists of several tests to detect and measure various compounds that pass through the urine. The purpose is to provide data on renal function useful for the physician to determine the patient's health status.

The examinations of this test consist of a physical examination that is performed based on an evaluation regarding its appearance, a chemical examination that is performed through reagent strips, and a microscopic examination of the urinary sediment that is obtained after a centrifugation, and if the doctor requires it, a urine culture is requested, the latter is not performed in the laboratory "El Carmen".

Urinalysis determinations are performed in the following chronological order.

12.8 Physical examination

This test involves the determination of color and appearance. It consists of direct observation of the urine in a clean, clear glass tube. Generally the color of urine is light yellow, but it can also have a slightly cloudy appearance due to decreased solubility or presence of crystals (urates, phosphates, calcium oxalate or uric acid), presence of cells (bacteria, erythrocytes, leukocytes, epithelial cells, etc.) or the existence of proteinuria or lipiduria. Where the urine normally possesses:

Color: yellow

Appearance: clean

In the event of an anomaly, they can be loaned:

Appearance:

•   Cloudy: Due to the presence of mucous substances, proteinuria, leukocytes, bacteriuria, precipitation of salts (amorphous phosphates in alkaline urine or urates in acid urine).

•   Opalescent appearance and yellowish-white color: Pus or urinary tract infection.

Color:

•   Reddish: Due to hematuria, hemoglobinuria, microglobinuria, beet ingestion, presence of amorphous urate crystals (not pathogenic).

•   Intense yellow, dark green to brownish: Bilirubin.

- Mahogany: Bile pigments or porphyrias.

- Dark brown, blackish: Alcaptonuria.

- Orange: Febrile state, treatment with rifampicin.

12.9 Chemical test

This test is included in the test strips and normally the reaction should be negative. If a positive reaction is observed, it is reported according to the intensity of the color developed. The urine is checked for density, pH, leukocytes, nitrites, protein, glucose, ketone bodies, urobilinogen, bilirubin and hemoglobin.

Urine test strips consist of small rigid plastic strips to which are attached small squares each impregnated with different reagents. If the compound present in the urine is present, when it comes into contact with the reagents it produces an easily observable color reaction. In addition to being positive (color change) or negative (no change), the different color intensities will give an idea of the amount of the analyzed compound present in the sample, allowing a semi-quantification of the compound.

Semiquantification is achieved by comparison of the developed color provided by the manufacturer as 5-6 squares with shades related to the concentration corresponding to each metabolite to be analyzed (28).

The parameters given by the test strip are normal if they are within the following ranges:

- Density: 1.005 - 1.0030 g/l

- pH 5.0 - 7.0

- Leukocytes: Negative

- Nitrites: Negative

- Proteins: < 10 mg/dL

- Glucose: Negative

- Ketone bodies: Negative

- Urobilinogen: Normal <1.0 mg/dL

- Bilirubin: Negative

- Hemoglobin: Negative

Density. Urine density provides information on the renal function of the concentration and dilution of urine, reflecting the weight and concentration of solutes. Its limits are permissible from 1.005 to 1.0030 g/l, when having a good hydration the density is less than 1.010 and when suffering from dehydration occurs when it is greater than 1.020 g/l. As a result, urine of varying tonicity can be obtained, with the aim of preserving the body water balance. Very concentrated urine (hypertonic with respect to plasma) appears when the kidney tends to conserve water due to a decrease in water intake, fever, gastrointestinal losses, diabetes, saccharin, etc. The use of diuretics, decrease, absence or lack of action of antidiuretic hormone, poor protein nutrition and diabetes insipidus are factors that result in the formation of dilute urine (hypotonic with respect to plasma).

pH. The strip contains a mixture of pH indicators that in contact with urine give a sharp gradation of colors, from orange (pH 5) to blue (pH 9). This parameter varies according to blood acid-base balance, renal function and, to a lesser extent, diet, drugs and sample exposure time.

The kidney is one of the organs that, together with the lung, is involved in the regulation of the concentration of H^+ in the extracellular fluid and does so mainly by regulating the concentration of plasma HCO_3. The normal excretion of H^+ gives mostly acidic characteristics to the urine, so the normal urinary pH range is between 5 and 7. Diets enriched in the consumption of fruits and vegetables give slightly alkaline urine, while the abundant intake of meats gives acidic urine. In pathological cases, acid reactions may be due to fever, metabolic acidosis, *E. coli* infection, diabetic ketoacidosis. Increased urinary pH is usually associated with alkaline diets, postprandial state, vomiting, urinary *Proteus spp.* infection, diuretic intake, respiratory alkalosis, distal renal tubular acidosis, etc.

Leukocytes. Granulocytes (neutrophils and eosinophils) are the only ones that possess the enzyme esterase in their cytoplasm, this enzyme reacts hydrolyzing the reagent of the strip making it change color, giving a violet colored product.

Nitrites. An amine is used which in an acid medium reacts with a diazonium salt, which reacts with a chromogen to form a pink color. The presence of bacteria in the urine is determined, more specifically enterobacteria such as *E. Coli* which have the particularity of reducing nitrates to nitrites.

Proteins. The strip contains an indicator that turns from yellow to green in the presence of protein. Normally no protein should be reported in the urine; protein excretion in the urine called proteinuria is a warning sign for the physician as it may mean probable damage at the glomerular or tubular level that will require specific studies for diagnosis. If the reaction is positive, the concentration should be determined in a 24-hour urine sample with a chemical method. Proteinuria is usually due to the following causes:

1.   Increase of normal and abnormal plasma proteins.

2.   Increased glomerular permeability.

3.   Decreased reabsorption of polypeptides and low-PM proteins that normally filter through the glomerulus.

4.   Hemodynamic alterations, including exercise, changes in position from decubitus to erect, fever, etc.

Glucose. Glucose, by the glucose oxidase present on the strip, is oxidized to gluconolactone and hydrogen peroxide, through the oxidase/peroxidase reaction. Hydrogen peroxide, in the presence of peroxidase also present on the strip, in turn oxidizes an indicator. The amount of product formed gives a range of color from yellow to green. The glucosuria reading should be zero because the filtered glucose is almost entirely reabsorbed.

Glucose filtered in the glomerulus is almost completely reabsorbed in the proximal convoluted tubule. This process is carried out by a membrane transporter that becomes saturated with glucose concentrations above 180 mg/dL in these circumstances the unreabsorbed glucose remains in luminal fluid and is excreted in the urine. The most common cause of glycosuria is uncontrolled diabetes mellitus. Since normal blood glucose is between 70 and 110 mg/dL, the presence of glycosuria is indicative of hyperglycemia although there are a number of entities characterized by abnormalities at the tubular level that present with intense glycosuria without the coexistence of hyperglycemia.

Ketone bodies. Only acetoacetate and acetone react with sodium nitroprusside and glycine in alkaline medium giving a violet complex. The β-hydroxybutyrate does not react. Ketone bodies are formed when the supply of fatty acids to the liver exceeds its capacity to utilize acetyl-CoA. They are then released into the blood from where they are taken up by aerobic organs for oxidation and energy production. Acetone is eliminated by breath, while acetoacetate and β-hydroxybutyrate are eliminated by urine. Their elimination only occurs in appreciable quantities when their synthesis is excessive, as occurs in decompensated diabetes mellitus, prolonged fasting and febrile processes.

In these cases ketonemia (presence in blood in high amounts) and ketonuria (presence in urine) are detected.

Urobilinogen. Urobilinogen reacts in acid medium with a diazonium salt, giving a red compound. Normal result: up to 1mg/dL. Urobilin and urobilinogen are increased by hemolysis and liver disorders.

Bilirubin. Bilirubin reacts with a diazonium salt in an acid medium, yielding a purplish-pink compound. The bilirubin present in urine is of the conjugated type, a water-soluble form that is filtered in the renal glomerulus, where it arrives after passing through the enterohepatic circulation. Bilirubin is present in the urine in cases of hemolytic jaundice and increased in cases of hepatitis, obstructive jaundice or pancreatic head neoplasms.

Hemoglobin. Hemoglobin has pseudo-peroxidative activity, so it is able to release O_2 from H_2O_2. In the test strips this oxygen production is coupled to the oxidation of the indicator benzidine (blue-green oxidized form). If the sample contains intact erythrocytes (hematuria), they are seen as isolated green dots or in clusters on the yellow background. If hemoglobinuria (free hemoglobin in urine) is present, the green color is homogeneous. These results should be corroborated by observation of the urine sediment. Normal result: negative (up to 5 erythrocytes per field).

13.2.1 Chemical test processing

1. To perform the chemical test set-up, the sample must be analyzed within 4 hours after its release.

2. The urine sample from the collection bottles should be slightly homogenized before being placed in the pre-labeled test tubes.

3. Take the test strip and use it as soon as possible, taking care to close the container immediately after removing the required number of strips.

4. Immerse the strip completely in the test tube containing fresh urine and immediately remove it from the container to prevent the reagents from dissolving.

5. When removing the urine strip, run the edge of the strip against the rim of the urine container to discard excess urine and hold the strip in a horizontal position in contact of the strip with an absorbent paper material.

6. Trigger the stopwatch for one minute to proceed with the interpretation of the test strips.

7. Use the corresponding color chart labeled on the tube, holding the strip close to the color chart.

8. If so, after centrifuging the samples, place two drops of sulfosalicylic acid to observe if the sample is cloudy, if so, it indicates the presence of proteins in the urine (29).

13.3 Microscopic examination

After performing the chemical test, we proceed to perform the methodology for the microscopic examination, which is described below:

•	The test tubes are centrifuged at a speed of 4000 rpm for a period of approximately 4 minutes.

•	At the end of the previous step, the supernatant is discarded from the test tube.

•	Resuspend 0.5 ml of the precipitant in order to homogenize the sample to be analyzed by tapping the test tube.

•	Place 50 µL of the urine precipitant on the slide using a micropipette plus a small drop of Sternheimer's staining dye.

•	Homogenize the urine sample and the dye and then place a coverslip, taking care that air bubbles do not tend to form.

•	Mount the sample in the microscope at 40X to proceed with the microscopic examination.

Urinary sediment:

•	Leukocytes: 0-5/40 x field

•	Erythrocytes: 0-2/ 40 x field

•	Epithelial cells: variable number

•	Cylinders: up to 2 hyaline/fields of 10 x

•	Crystals: variable quantity

Urine sediment microscopic examination is a routine diagnostic test that is performed primarily to determine the health status of the patient to detect and evaluate the presence of microscopic form elements and particles of the urinary tract that make up part of the urine, such as leukocytes, erythrocytes, epithelial cells, bacteria, casts, crystals, tumor cells; where all these factors are indicative of renal or urinary tract disorders. The value of this analysis depends on the standardized method and the experience of the operator who performs it.

The urinary sediment is usually practically empty, although occasionally cells from the urinary tract and even from the external genitalia may be observed, as well as isolated erythrocytes or leukocytes, crystals, amorphous salts or mucus filaments, the rest of the elements being of probable pathological origin. The pathological components most often observed are quite unspecific and are evidenced in various diseases of the urinary tract.

Sediment entities that should be identified using microscopic examination of the sediment include the following:

- Epithelial cells

- Leukocytes

- Erythrocytes

- Cylinders

- Bacteria

- Crystals

- Mucoid networks

13.3.1 Epithelial cells

0 Cells of the urethral epithelium.

They are the most common cells found within the urethral tissue, they present an epithelium with three layers of cells that are recognized morphologically because they change from one to another gradually as they mature in their ascent through the tissue. It presents a flat stratified epithelium where its synonyms would also be squamous and pavement. A low to moderate cell count is considered to be within normal limits, but an abundance of numerous cells may be a sign of medical problems such as urinary tract infection, candida infection, kidney disease or cancer.

- basal cells: They measure about 20 to 30 µm in diameter, have an oval cytoplasm, round to oval nucleus of 15 to 18 µm with a thin nuclear membrane, a uniform chromatin and no nucleolus.

- intermediate cells: They measure about 50 to 60 µm in diameter, their cytoplasm is irregular and slightly elongated, with an oval nucleus of about 10 µm, a thin nuclear membrane with a uniform chromatin and no nucleolus.

- Superficial cells: They measure about 60 to 70 µm in diameter, have a polygonal cytoplasm with many irregular sides or very thin flat cytoplasm (may show some small granules) and a small pyknotic nucleus.

Urethral cell morphology

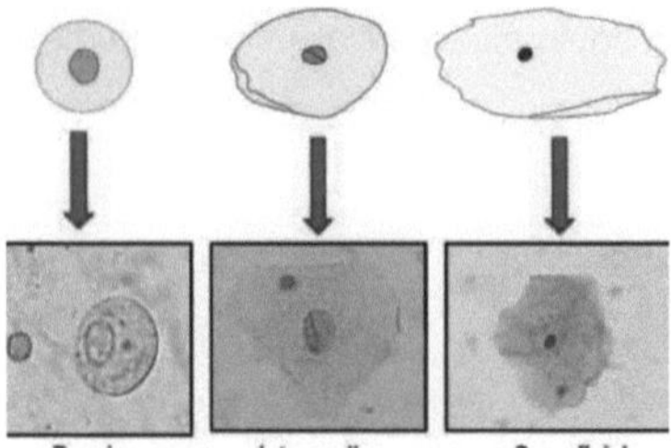

Figure 28. Cells of the urethral epithelium.

0 Cells of bladder, ureters and renal pelvis.

They present a transitional epithelium or urothelium. It is also a stratified epithelium with three recognizable layers. They are identified by the fact that they are smaller than those of the urethral epithelium, they are rounded with a "tail" and their nucleus is larger and rounder.

•	Basal: 15 to 20 μm in greatest diameter, with a scanty cytoplasm with caudal extension, an elliptical nucleus with a thick membrane, granular chromatin and a nucleolus present.

•	Intermediate: 30 to 50 μm in diameter with a more extensive cytoplasm, the shape changes from oval to geometric, with straight and long sides, usually 5 to 6-sided, with a round nucleus, thick membrane and granular chromatin with the presence of a nucleolus.

•	Superficial: They measure from 60 to 80 μm, have an extensive cytoplasm of geometric shape, generally hexagonal, with straight and long edges, may have two or more round nuclei, with thick membrane and granular chromatin and presence of nucleolus.

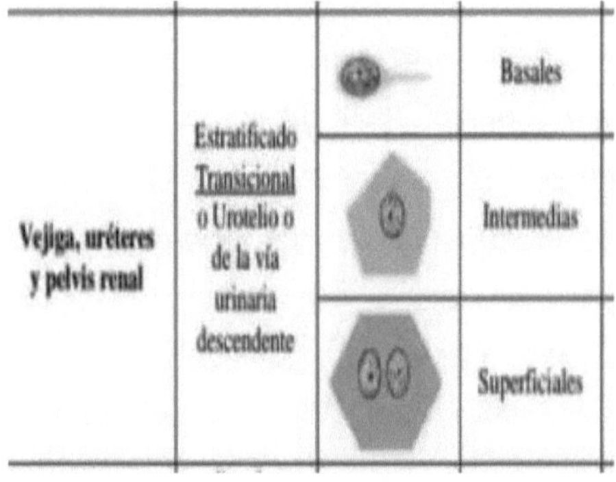

Vejiga, uréteres y pelvis renal	Estratificado Transicional o Urotelio o de la vía urinaria descendente		Basales
			Intermedias
			Superficiales

Figure 29. Cells of bladder ureters and renal pelvis.

0 Renal tubules (renal cells)

86

The renal tubules are formed by a simple cubic epithelium. When the cells are detached they take a spherical shape and are usually found individually. They are cells presenting granulations, where their nucleus is very large and round and difficult to visualize. The presence of these cells suggests the existence of a nephrotic syndrome. Their characteristics are as follows.

- They measure 14 to 16 µm in diameter, their cytoplasm is granular spherical, the nucleus is eccentric and round, has a thick membrane of granular chromatin with the presence of a nucleolus.

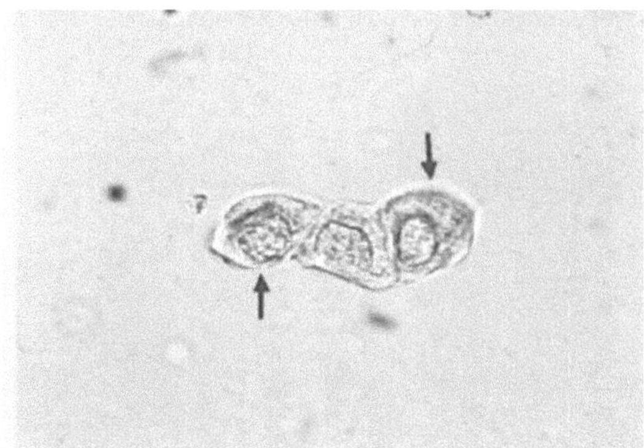

Figure 30. Cells of the renal tubule.

0 Neoplastic cells

Most urinary tract neoplasms are located in the transitional epithelium of the bladder to the renal pelvis, beginning with papillary hyperplasia and increased cell growth with incomplete maturation. These cells have a strong resemblance to renal tubular cells, but occur in a three-dimensional formation resembling a cluster of grapes. They can also be found as flat, plaque-like clusters of cells that commonly have very little cytoplasm and are malignant. The last common presentation in these cases is that of spindle or elongated cells, with an eccentric nucleus and very long and thin cytoplasm. All of them lose differentiation of the cytoplasm but retain the nuclear features mentioned for normal transitional cells.

13.3.2 Leukocytes

The chemist reports the approximate number of leukocytes per field, which are visible cells larger than erythrocytes and smaller than epithelial cells, with the presence of segmented nuclei and granulations. When observing a urinary sediment of a healthy person, up to 5 leukocytes per field can be detected without any pathological significance.

In women it should be noted that the leukocytes found may be of vaginal origin, especially if accompanied by a large number of flat epithelial cells, so the study of midstream urine may be of great value in clarifying this issue.

When reporting the results, a normal parameter is considered when 0 to 5 leukocytes per field are found. And it is defined as leukocyturia when a higher number of leukocytes passes into the categories of moderate and abundant and/or very abundant leukocytes per field. In any case, a high number of leukocytes in the urine is a sign that you are probably going through an inflammatory process in the kidney or urinary tract and there is a possibility of acute or chronic pyelonephritis, urethritis, mycosis, prostatitis, cystitis, pyelitis and tuberculosis.

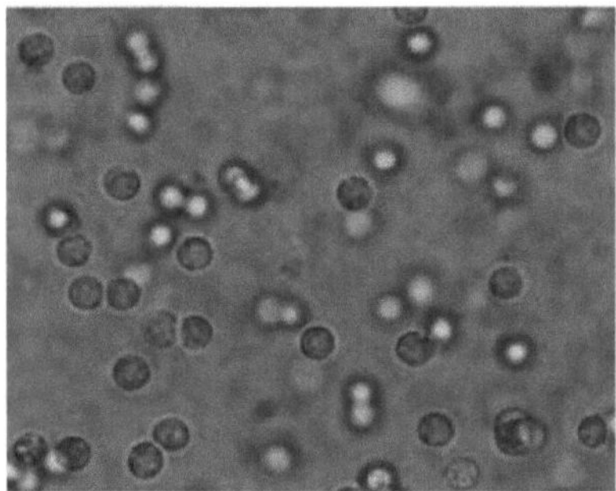

Figure 31. Leukocytes in urinary sediment.

13.3.3 Erythrocytes

Erythrocytes are eliminated in a small part in the urine, even in normal persons, under normal conditions approximately 0 to 2 hematocytes per field can be observed. Similarly, in the same term above, ranging from scanty, moderate or abundant cells per field are reported.

On microscopic examination they are identified as round discs of faint reddish-yellow color, with double contour. The membrane of erythrocytes is too permeable, that is why they contain different conditions of solutes present in urine, erythrocytes undergo morphological changes in their shape and size, depending on the factors based on the osmotic gradient of solutes present in urine, so erythrocytes can be observed swollen, crenated or of normal size. In hypotonic urine erythrocytes swell and in urine with hypertonic solutions erythrocytes wrinkle. The morphology of the hematocytes can reveal the glomerular or postglomerular origin of the hematuria.

In itself, an elevated number of red blood cells in the urine called hematuria may indicate an infection present in the lower urinary tract, renal injury such as calculi, bladder cancer, prostate problems, etc. (30).

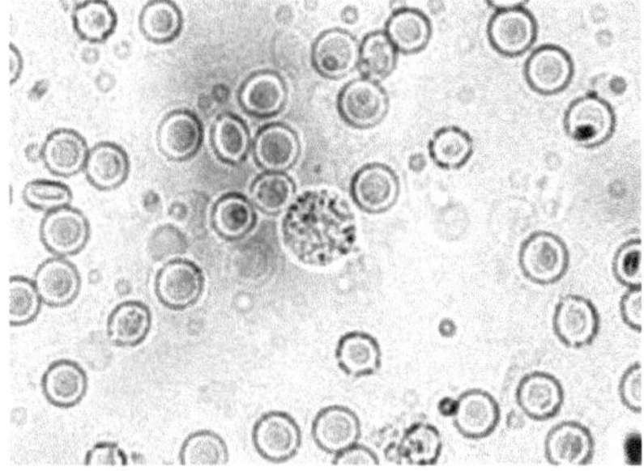

Figure 32. Erythrocytes in urinary sediment.

13.3.4 Cylinders

The presence of casts almost always indicates the presence of renal disease, although evidence of some of them (hyaline and granular) can be found in healthy people who made great physical efforts, and sometimes in dehydration and fever.

Cylinders are usually caused by the fact that urine, under conditions of acidification, maximum urine concentration and its maximum range point, causes longitudinal structure-forming proteins to precipitate. Similarly, when urine tends to be in very dilute conditions, the cylinders tend to dissolve. There are different types of proteins.

Hyaline cylinder

It is composed of a high molecular weight protein that is produced and eliminated in very small quantities under normal conditions. These cylinders are homogeneous, colorless, transparent and refract little light, making them easy to miss.

This cylinder can be found in isolated form in healthy persons or under the administration of diuretics such as furosemide, in conditions of nephrotic syndrome the number of cylinders increases drastically. Hyaline casts with cellular inclusions (erythrocytes, leukocytes, tubular epithelium) are detected, which determines the presence of disease in glomerulopathies.

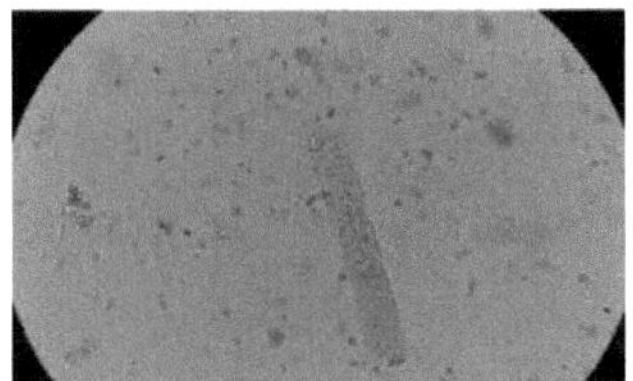

Granular cylinders

Sometimes they can appear in healthy and sick people, although their presence is related to acute and chronic diseases of the kidney such as glomerulonephritis and is slightly associated with pyelonephritis. They are usually larger than hyaline and present granular inclusions, besides this type of cylinders has a higher refraction of light that favors its visualization. A mixture of hyaline and granular casts can be observed.

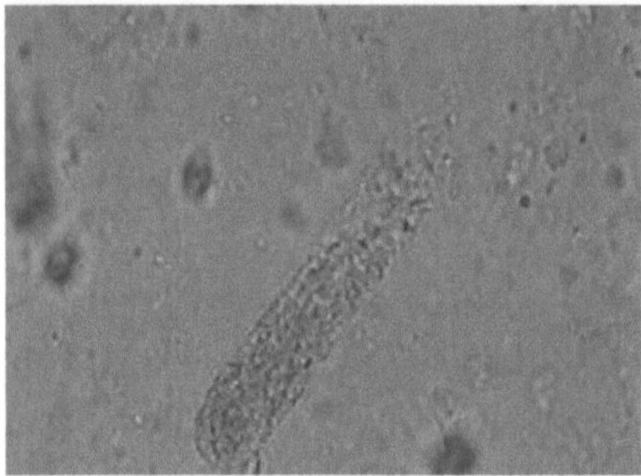

Figure 34. Granular cylinder.

Waxy cylinders

They are usually wider than the hyaline ones, show a higher refraction of light, which makes them not easy to miss, projecting a slightly yellowish hue. It presents notches, breaks or fine indentations that are observed on the edges of the cylinder. Its presence always indicates a severe chronic kidney disease in a patient with advanced chronic renal failure, but sometimes it can be observed in the recovery phase of diuresis after a period of suspension of urine secretion.

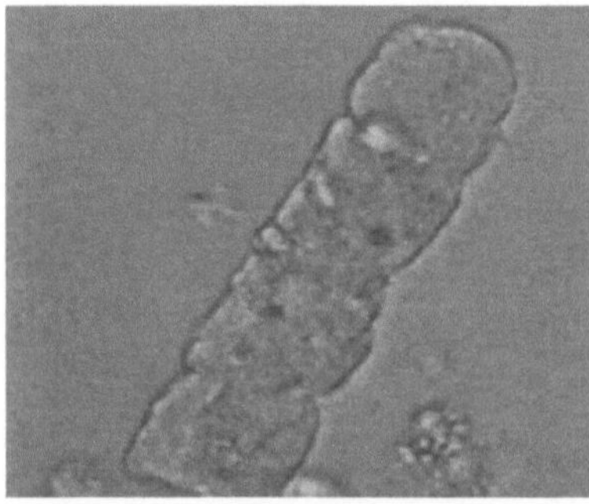

Figure 35. Ceric cylinder.

Epithelial cylinders

They are composed of desquamated tubular epithelium. Their presence is especially appreciated in the recovery phase of diuresis after acute renal failure due to ischemic or toxic tubular necrosis. They are rare.

Cylinders with lipidic inclusions: They differ from the epithelial ones by the inclusion of fat droplets in the tubular cells. They are observed in the course of a nephrotic syndrome.

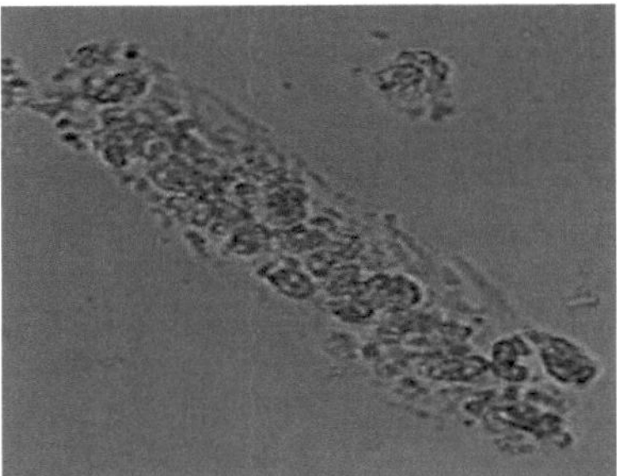

Figure 36. Epithelial cylinder.

Erythrocyte cylinders

As the name implies, they are composed of swollen erythrocytes that adhere to a hyaline ground substance. They are identified under the microscope by the color between red, yellow, brown, and colorless. They always indicate the renal origin of the hematuria and therefore it is a very valuable finding. They appear in glomerular lesions, mainly in acute and chronic glomerulonephritis, lupus nephropathy, panarteritis, nodosa, bacterial endocarditis associated with glomerulonephritis.

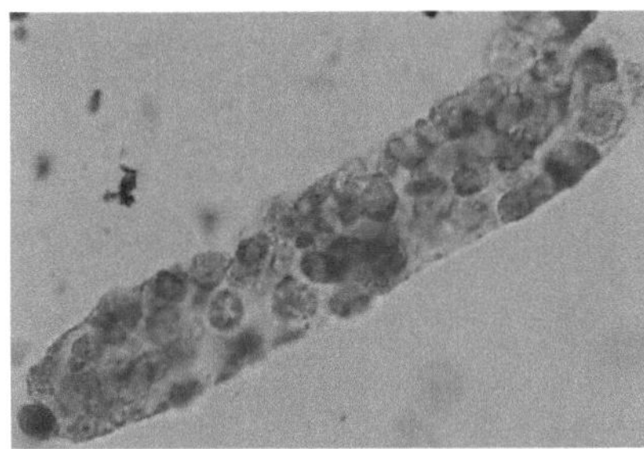

Figure 37. Erythrocyte cylinders.

Leukocyte cylinder

These casts are produced when an intense exudation of leukocytes occurs at the same time that proteins are eliminated by the tubule. Their presence is of fundamental importance because it shows that the inflammation is of renal origin, almost always due to pyelonephritis and glomerulonephritis.

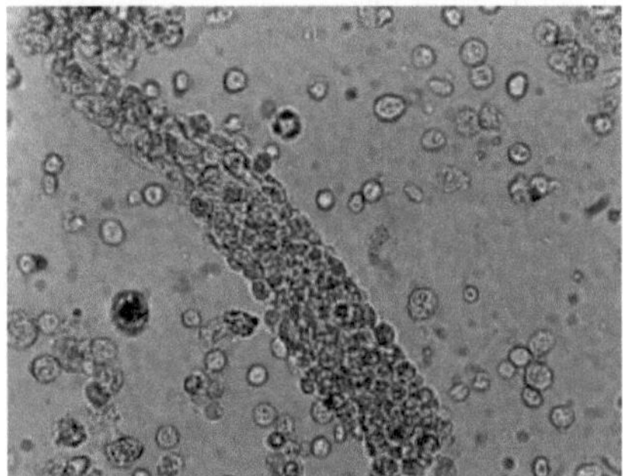

Figure 38. Leukocyte cylinder.

13.3.5 Crystals

Crystals can adopt multiple forms depending on the chemical compound and the pH at which the urine is found. The presence of crystals in the urine is called crystalluria, which in some cases has diagnostic significance depending on the compound of which they are formed. One of the main characteristics of the urine is the coolness, which under polarized light will be called birefringence, this being positive if the crystal appears in a blue tone or negative if it appears in a yellow tone. Crystalluria and there are several methods to help distinguish it, such as polarized light. In acid urine amorphous urate, uric acid and calcium oxalate crystals are observed, while in alkaline urine phosphate crystals are observed. (31) Among the most frequent crystals in urine we have:

Urates

They are found in amorphous form in acidic or neutral urine or in the form of a cylinder, which can lead to confusion. When they are eliminated in large quantities, they are recognized macroscopically as a red-brown precipitate (brick dust). They are basically dark granulations with a yellow-orange or pinkish color. They are of no diagnostic importance but may be present in febrile and gouty states.

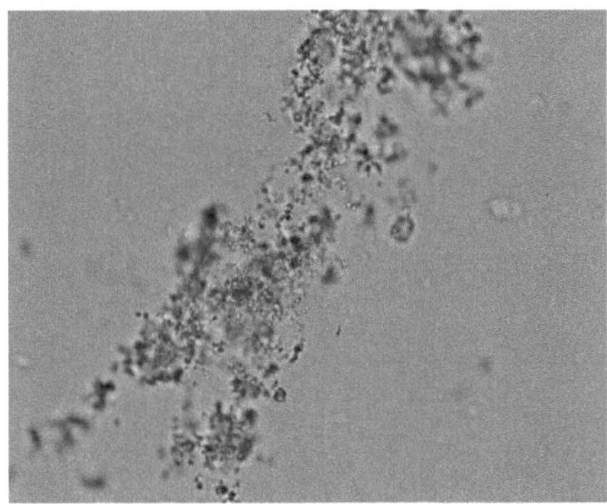

Uric acid

They appear in acid urine and can take various forms (rhomboidal squares, rectangular or hexagonal, rosettes, barrels, etc.). They have a reddish yellow color. They are frequent in concentrated urine, appear in fever, gout and tumor lysis, urinary tract calculi, but are not usually of great interest.

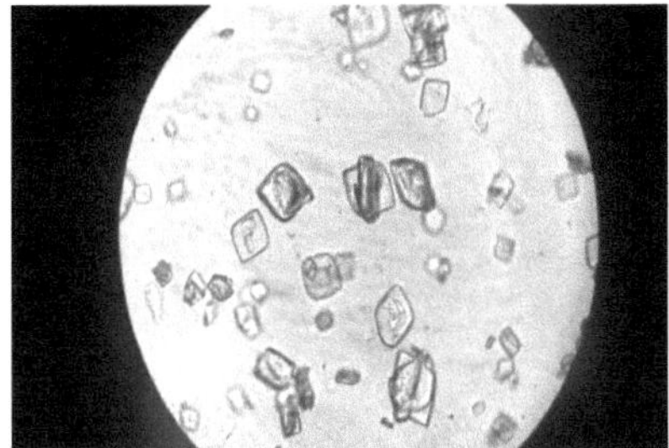

Figure 40. Uric acid crystals.

Calcium oxalate

It appears in urine with acid or neutral pH, are colorless crystals and very birefringent. Characteristic is their form in envelopes or in octahedral forms of variable size. They occur very frequently after the ingestion of food rich in oxalate such as tomatoes, garlic, oranges, or asparagus. They also appear in diabetes or hepatopathies.

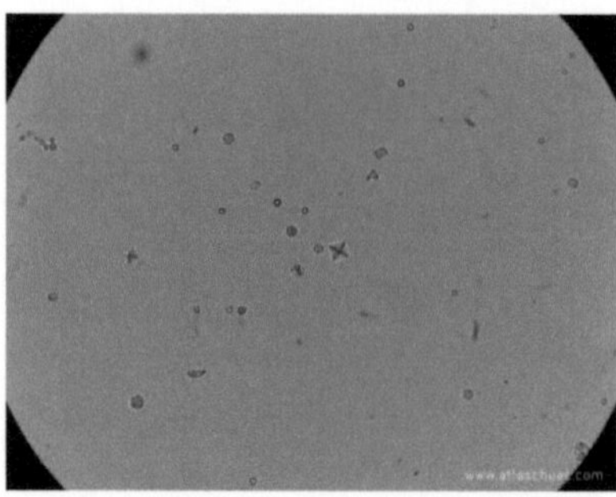

Figure 41. Calcium oxalate crystals.

Calcium sulfate

They are observed as long, thin, colorless prisms or needles. They are rare and are only detected in urine with very acidic pH.

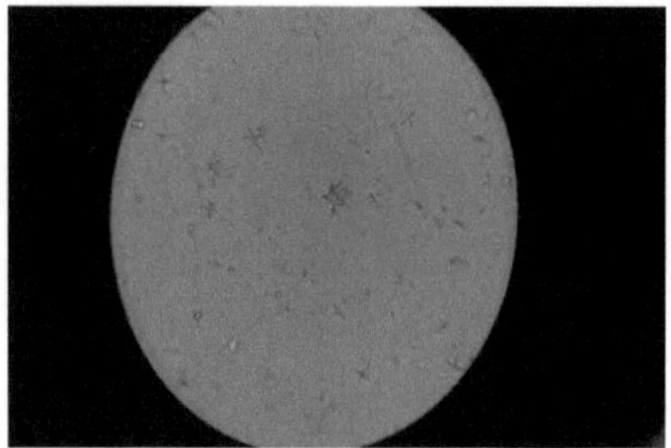

Figure 42. Calcium sulfate crystals.

Leucine and tyrosine

They usually appear together as a result of severe liver disease or tissue necrosis and are very rare. They are found in acidic urine and have yellowish tones.

The appearance of tyrosine (pink) is not very recurrent, it has the form of very fine needles and its color ranges from colorless to brownish yellow, they are very refrigent and appear in groups or clusters. Leucine (brown) forms spheres in whose interior concentric concentrations appear, they are highly refrigent and appear yellowish or brownish.

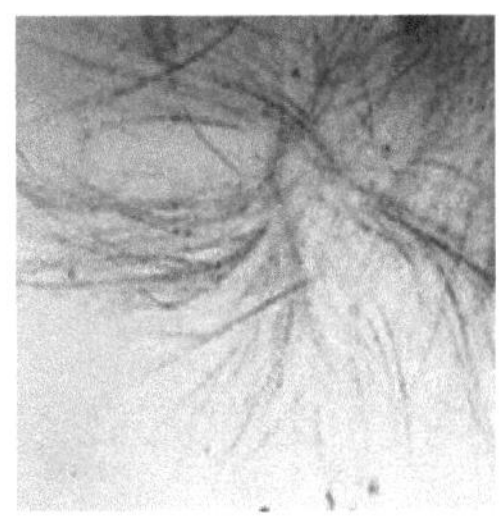

Figure 43. Tyrosine needles.

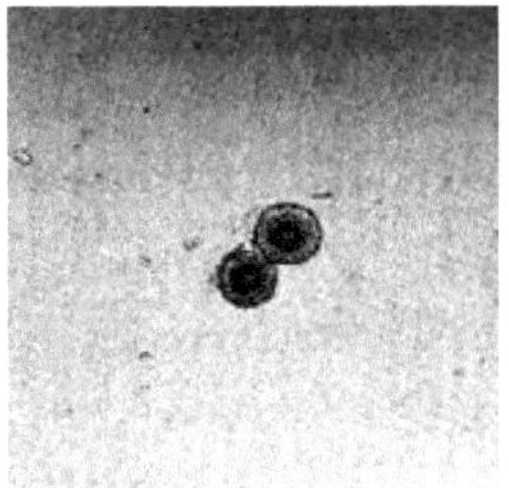

Figure 44. Leucine spheres.

Magnesium ammonium phosphate or triple phosphate phosphate

They are seen as colorless, three- to six-sided prism-like forms with a "coffin lid" appearance and are present in alkaline urine. They are birefringent to polarized light which helps in their identification. They appear as a consequence of ammonia fermentation in cases of marked bacteriuria, indicating infection by bacteria such as *Proteus, Morganella, ureaplasma* and *Corynebacterium urealyticum.*

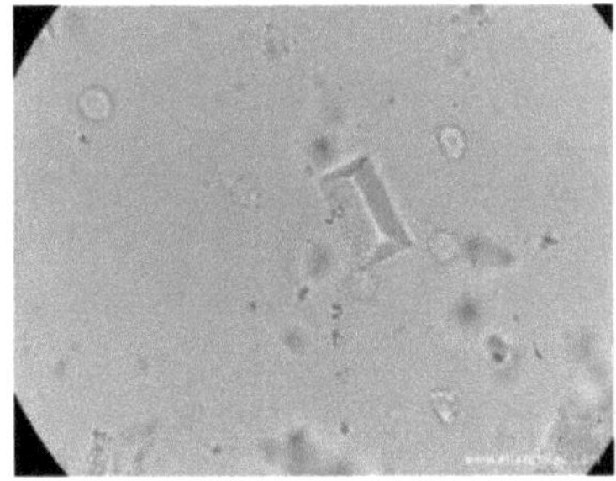

Figure 45. Ammonium phosphate.

Cystine

They are detected in acidic urine as colorless and very fine hexagonal squares with high refraction. They are observed in cystinuria, a congenital disorder of cystine tubular reabsorption; they appear in patients with hereditary metabolic disorders.

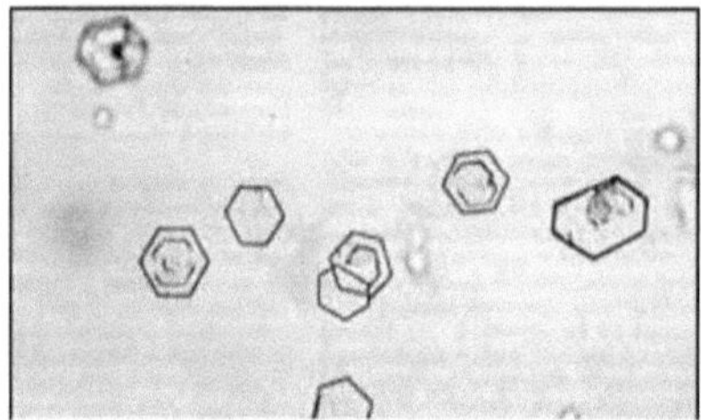

Figure 46. Cystine

Cholesterol crystals

They can be found in acidic or neutral urine, although they are not very common in urine sediment. They are observed as flat transparent sheets with notched edges or in the form of transparent plates or prisms cleaved regularly or irregularly. They are often found forming a film on the surface of the urine. They are related to pathologies of the nephrotic syndrome and predominate in chyluria (passage of lymph into the urine), where there is rupture of the lymphatic vessels of the renal pelvis. They are not found in healthy individuals.

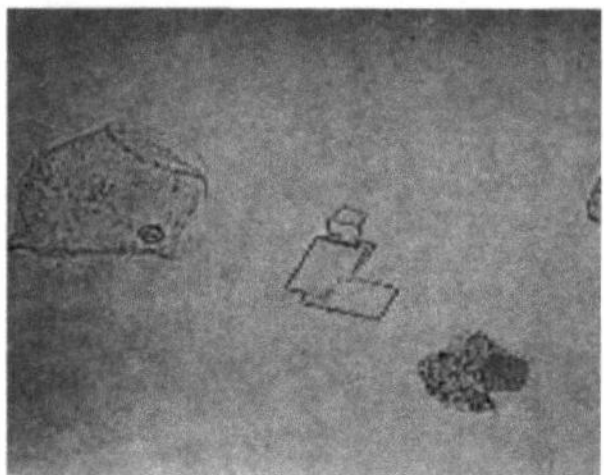

Figure 47. Cholesterol crystals.

Ammonium urate

They are the only urates found in alkaline urines. They are yellow-brown in color and have various spherical shapes grouped with a radial striation in long spicules with irregular edges or without them.

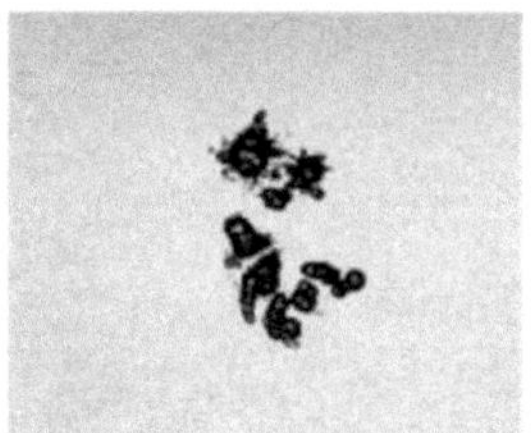

Figure 48. Ammonium urate.

Amorphous phosphate crystals

They appear in alkaline or neutral urine. They are found as clusters of small granules but have no clinical significance. They are found abundantly in patients with calcium phosphate lithiasis.

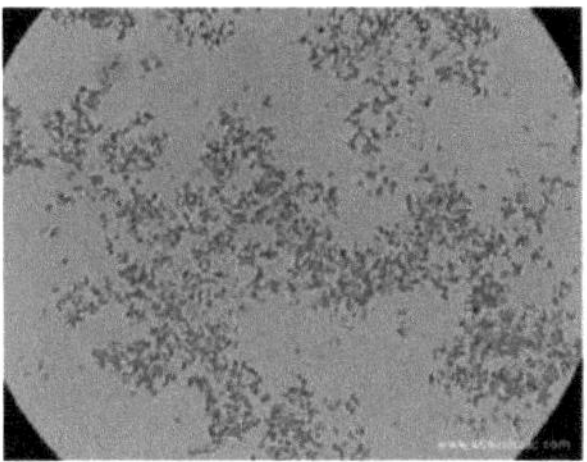

Figure 49. Amorphous phosphate crystals

13.3.6 Bacteria

There is no presence of bacteria in the kidneys or bladder. Under normal conditions, urine is free of bacteria, but it can be contaminated by bacteria present in the urethra or vagina. Bacteria are found in the form of cocci or bacilli and differ from amorphous salts by their spontaneous mobility. They have weak birefringence, are generally apinate and often produce streaks and are considerably smaller in size than erythrocytes. When a urine sample is collected correctly and in a sterile manner and contains a large number of bacteria and is accompanied by many leukocytes, a urinary tract infection is very likely to be found.

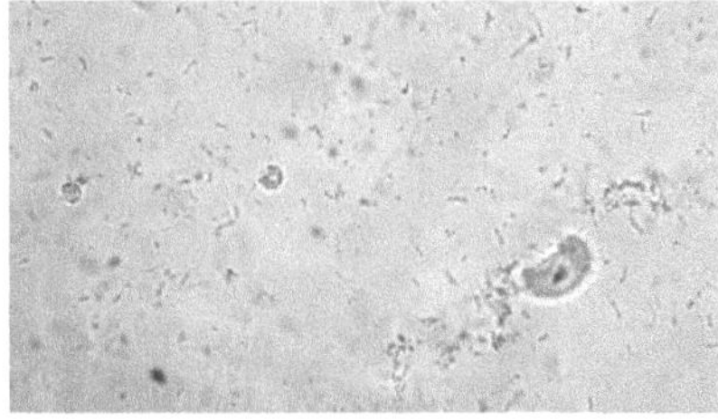

Figure 50. Bacteria in the form of lines.

13.3.7 Mushrooms

Fungi are colorless, oval-shaped structures, somewhat smaller than erythrocytes. Confusion can be avoided by considering that fungi are usually of variable size and often have extensions. These evaginations often give rise to tubular or filamentous structures (hyphae), which can be recognized by the characteristic transverse septa. When many of these hyphae accumulate and branch we speak of mycelium.

It is common to find them in urine in patients with metabolic diseases such as diabetes mellitus. In glycosuria it is frequent to observe fungi and in general these are patients with weakened defenses; *Candida albicans* plays a fundamental role causing candidiasis.

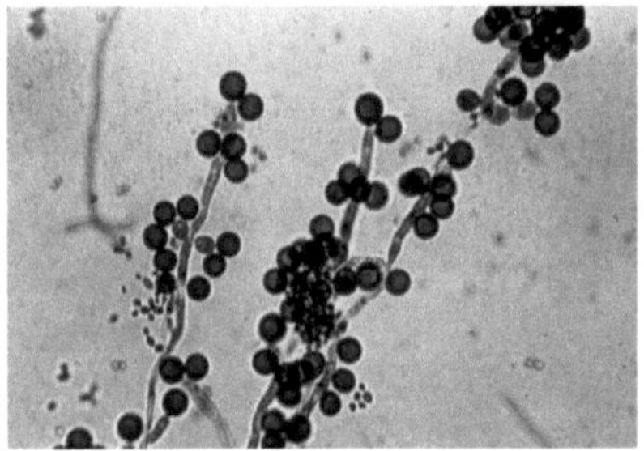

Figure 51. *Candida albicans* fungus.

13.3.8 Mucus filament

Mucus filaments are very frequent in urine, especially when it is cooled. Their length is sometimes so great that they can even be recognized macroscopically. However, they are usually irregular filaments of varying length, whether long, thin or undulating, which are only visible in dim light. Sometimes epithelial cells, leukocytes, erythrocytes and even crystals hang from these mucous filaments. These structures are normally found in small quantities, there is pathological significance when they are very abundant in infammation or irritation of the urinary tract, they have no pathological significance.

Figure 52. Mucus filament

13.3.9 Fat droplets

Fat droplets in urine are round, highly refrigent structures that have a black appearance when examined under magnification. Because of their high birefringence and variable size they can be easily differentiated from erythrocytes.

Fat droplets as well as cells or casts with fat droplet inclusions are seen in nephrotic syndrome.

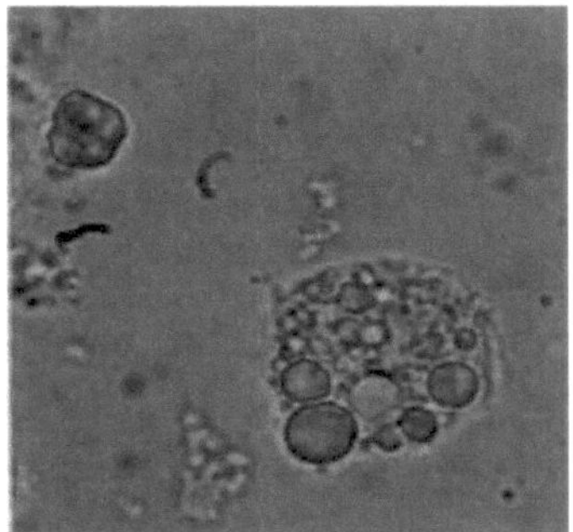

Figure 53. Fat droplets.

14. Quality control

In order to detect and correct analytical deficiencies within the laboratory, it is necessary to perform quality control tests to ensure the reliability of the results issued.

Quality control in the clinical laboratory is a system designed to increase the probability that each result reported by the laboratory is valid and can be used with confidence by the physician to make a diagnostic or therapeutic decision. Quality control procedures work by detecting analytical errors. The quality tests that are performed during all analytical phases depend on each sample.

Some samples are rejected prior to analysis due to various factors such as inadequate identification, incorrect collection material used, hemolysis, or improper transport. When this occurs, a determination is made to re-sample under appropriate conditions.

In the case of reagents and equipment, in order to evaluate the reagents. Sets of tests are carried out under a procedure in which a technique is performed that indicates whether the reagents and equipment are in optimal conditions to continue to be used and give a reliable result.

Factors that may cause a variation in the results may be due to environmental conditions, the temperature at which the reagents are handled (optimum from 8 to 0 °c), the time the reagents have been exposed since they were taken out of the packaging, the expiration date, the service performed on the equipment, any batch or reagent change, the calibration of the equipment before use, among others.

The quality control management of the automated system requires a previous preparation before its proper use, which consists of a maintenance and a process that is necessary to verify an excellent performance of the instrument, while evaluating the conditions of the reagents used.

To have a cherry on top of the results in the equipment. Statistical parameters and a series of controls will indicate the precision and accuracy with which we are reporting the results.

In blood chemistry equipment, for example, a control sample is used as if it were that of a patient with a precisely assigned value, which has already been tested according to the reference method. Known controls or standards are used for this purpose, which should be 3 different levels (low, normal and high) in order to establish a predictable mathematical relationship between the true value of the analyte and the instrument result, thereby confirming the accuracy of the instrument by comparing the instrument result against an acceptable standard value.

Cases may occur in which a run is rejected, so the test should be repeated, if after that the values are not corrected, the possible causes of error should be investigated, it may be due to deterioration of the reagent, problems with the pump tubing or light source, if after checking these details the error persists, look for a simple fault in the equipment, if after this the error continues it is advisable to notify the specialized technical support service of the instrument supplier.

All the instruments on which the tests are performed must be properly managed for maintenance and electronic stability. The general technique to implement the quality control of the equipment consists of:

1. Give the equipment a start-up that is in charge of performing a flushing and purging of the corresponding reagents in hoses and pipes; voltage readings, equipment pressures, etc.

2. Pass the controls (in the case of blood chemistry) that allow to supervise the stability of the electrical processing and flow evaluation systems used to measure volume, conductivity and laser light scattering. Once it is observed that the values obtained from the controls are within the limits, the instrument is considered to be well maintained and working properly.

3. At the end of the reading of the last sample, the equipment requires washing and purging in order to avoid the formation of plugs, dragging traces of reagents or analyte. This avoids contamination of future samples.

For the serology area, it consists basically of frequent day-to-day monitoring of the expiration date of the reagents used, in addition to monitoring them in the warehouse area.

Much about quality control is linked to the conditions in which patients are asked to collect their samples, in the case of urine, it is important that they are processed within 4 hours; and for urine and pharyngeal samples they are refrigerated and stored at a temperature of 2°C, for a period of no more than 24 hours. They are then taken to the specialized laboratory that will process them.

Every day in the morning, the temperature of the refrigerator that stores all the reagents in the laboratory is checked (with a thermometer). The temperature fluctuations are always noted down on a sheet of paper, taking care that it is always between 2 and 8°C.

15. Handling of the RPBI

All biohazardous biological-infectious waste is separated in the laboratory according to its physical and biological-infectious characteristics, as indicated in Mexican Official Standard 087-ECOL-SSA1-2002. Biological-infectious hazardous waste should not be mixed with any other type of municipal or hazardous waste.

Swabs with stained or dried blood, glassware used in the laboratory, urine and feces samples are not considered infectious biological hazardous waste.

Once the samples are finished, they are refrigerated for a period of one week, in order to have a sample available in case a patient requires an additional test and there is no need to perform another blood collection. Vacutainer tubes that are stored in the refrigerator are placed in red plastic bags.

Sharps waste such as disposable syringe needles and lancets are deposited in rigid red polypropylene containers. It is recommended that the containers be placed approximately 1 meter or 1.5 meters away from where the procedure is being performed. To avoid accidental needle sticks, needles should be discarded uncapped. If recapping is necessary, it should be done on a solid surface, avoiding the two-handed technique.

Once the plastic containers and bags reach 80% of their capacity, the waste is transported to another laboratory where a specialized company transports it to a final site where it is given an adequate final treatment.

16. Regulations

Mexican Official Standard NOM-087-2002-SSA1-ECOL environmental protection-environmental health-biological-infectious hazardous waste-classification and handling specifications.

Mexican Official Standard NOM-007- SSA3-2011 for the organization and operation of clinical laboratories.

17. Conclusion

The role played by the Pharmaceutical Chemist Biologist in the laboratory involves several factors, which at certain stages, if not carried out, could jeopardize the health, credibility, professionalism and compromise the health of patients.

In the case of the application of the regulations carried out in the laboratory, it indicates the guidelines that must be followed for the correct handling of the samples, the conditions in which they must work and the management of the residues that are generated. The results are completely reliable and of good quality.

The application of knowledge in the laboratory area is crucial to give the best interpretation to the results that are issued by the laboratory, and made available to the physician to rule out or confirm a certain diagnosis.

Bibliography

1. **Buitrago, José Manuel Gonzalez De.** *Clinical laboratory techniques and methods.* Barcelona Spain : El sevier Masson, 2010. pàg. 4. ISBN.

2. **Wshintong C. Ween, Allen, janda.** *koneman Diagnostico Microbiológico Texto y Atlas en color.* sexta. Buenos Aires Argentina : Panamericana, 2008. pg. 72. ISBN.

3. *BD Diagnósticos Sistemas Preanaliticos Product catalog for vein, arterial and urine sample collection.* Mexico DF : s.n., 2012.

4. **Vacuette.** *Blood filtration system handling recommendations.* 2011.

5. **Garcia, Ma. del Carmen Silva.** *Technician specialist in primary care laboratory of the Catalân Institute of Health.* Spain : MAD S.L, 2006. ISBN.

6. **Argüelles, Gilleromo J. Ruiz.** *Fundamentals of Hematology.* Mexico : Medica panamericana, 2009.

7. *Determiantion of reference intervals of hematological biomethylation in Mexican population.* **Piedra, Gabriela Olay.** 4, Mexico : Rev Latinoamer Patol Clin, 2012, Vol. 5.

8. *Semiology of hematological cytometia.* **Monroy, Rafael Hurtado.** 4, Mexico : Revista de Facultad de Medicina de la UNAM, 2010, Vol. 53.

9. **Nora, Brenden and Maria, Aguirre.** *Hemoglobin. Chair of Biochemistry, Faculty of Medicine, UNNE.* 2008.

10. **Montalvo, José Eduardo.** *Blood tissue and hematopoiesis.* Mexico : s.n.

11. *Theoretical review of cell biology and medical histology.* Mexico : s.n., 2012.

12. **Nieto, Anabella Quintana.** *Importance of blood biometry in medical practice.* Mexico City : Universidad Nacional Autónoma de México, 2008.

13. **Guyton, Arthur C.** *Treatise on Medical Physiology.* Spain : El sevier saunders, 2011. ISBN.

14. *Mean platelet volume and its significance in medical practice.* **Esper, Raúl Carrillo and Córdova, Dulce Maria Carrillo.** 1, Mexico : Rev Invest MedSurMex, 2013, Vol. 20.

15. **Rodak, Bernadette F.** *Hematology Fundamentals and Clinical Applications.* Buenos Aires : Medica Panamericana, 2004. ISBN.

16. *ABO blood group system.* **Garcia, Carlos Alberto Arbelàez.** 7-8, Bogotà : Mèdica Colombiana, 2009, Vol. 15.

17. **Duboscq, Cristina.** *Automation in Hemostasis.* Argentina : Fundacion Bioquimica Argentina, 2012.

18. **M., Gilberto Angel.** *Interpretación ciinica del Laboratorio.* bogotà : Mèdica Internacional, 2006. ISBN.

19. **Pagana, Kathleen Deska.** *Guia de pruebas diagnósticas y de laboratorio.* Spain : Elsevier, 2008. ISBN.

20. *Urea cycle disorders.* **Marián Carretero Colomer.** 9, Barcelona : Esteve, 2004, Vol.

23.

21. *Renal function studies: glomerular and tubular function. Urine analysis.* **Bibao, Itziar Castano.** 17-30, Pamplona : El Sevier, 2009, Vol. 2.

22. *The hyperuracemic patient.* **Aragón, Sagrario Martin.** 11, Madrid : Nutrifarmacia, 2006, Vol.

20.

23. **Rivera, José Maria Teijón y Pertierra, Armando Garrido.** *Fundamentals of Metabolic Biochemistry.* Madrid : Tebar, 2006. ISBN.

24. **Gerique, José Antonio Gómez.** *C-reactive protein as a marker of any type of inflammation.* Madrid : Biohealth Preveattion, 2006.

25. **Francisco Javier López Longo, Carlos Manuel Gonzàlez Fernàndez.** *Antibodies in rheumatoid arthritis.* Madrid : Revista Espanpla de Reumatologia Suplementos, 2002.

26. **Morales, T.M.Rodrigo Colina.** *Technical procedure for the serological diagnosis of syphilis.* Chile : Instituto de Salud Pùblica, 2015.

27. *Acquired Immunodeficiency Syndrome HIV/AIDS.* Chile : Ministry of Health, 2010. ISBN.

28. **Campos, Laura Delgado.** *Analysis of a urine sample by the laboratory.* 2011.

29. **Otegui, Vicente de Maria y Campos.** *Guia pràctica para la estandarización del procesamiento y examen de las muestras de urina.* s.l. : Bio-Rad Laboratories.

30. **Sabine Althof, Joachim Kindler.** *The Urinary Sediment.* Madrid : Panamericana, 2006. ISBN.

31. **Joaquin Cano Medina, Regina Bano.** *Current issues in urinalysis.* Malagà : Fesitess Andalucia, 2011. ISBN.

32. *J. M. Arribas Castrollo, Emilio Vllina.* *Hematologia Clinica Temas de Patologia Mèdica. University of Oviedo : Textos universitarios ediuno, 2005. ISBN.*

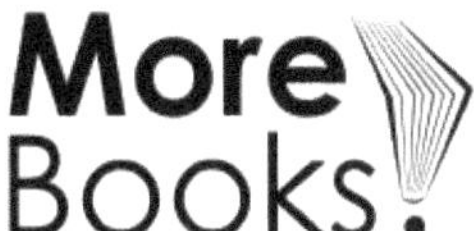

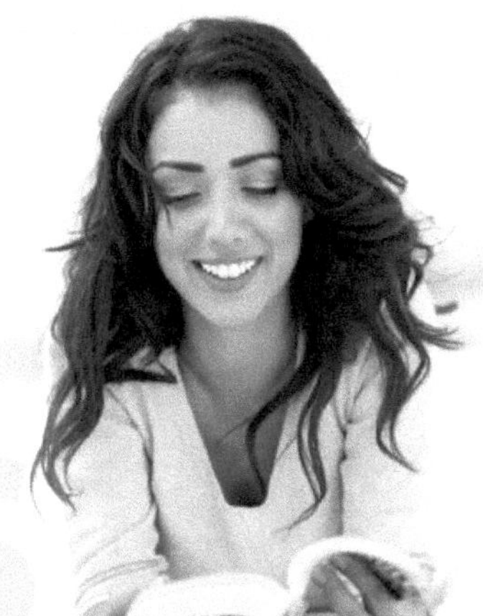

I want morebooks!

Buy your books fast and straightforward online - at one of world's fastest growing online book stores! Environmentally sound due to Print-on-Demand technologies.

Buy your books online at
www.morebooks.shop

Kaufen Sie Ihre Bücher schnell und unkompliziert online – auf einer der am schnellsten wachsenden Buchhandelsplattformen weltweit! Dank Print-On-Demand umwelt- und ressourcenschonend produziert.

Bücher schneller online kaufen
www.morebooks.shop

info@omniscriptum.com
www.omniscriptum.com

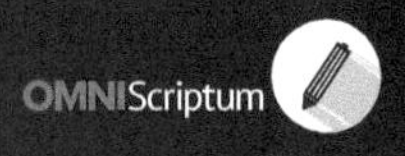

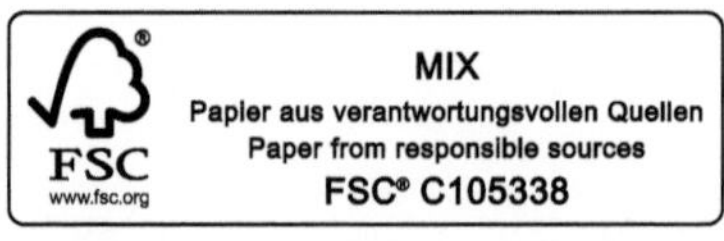

Printed by Books on Demand GmbH, Norderstedt / Germany